DR. MAO'S

SECRETS of LONGEVITY
COOKBOOK

EAT to THRIVE, LIVE LONG, and BE HEALTHY

DR. MAO SHING NI

PHOTOGRAPHY BY PHILIP DIXON

Andrews McMeel
Publishing, LLC

Kansas City • Sydney • London

Andrews McMeel Publishing, LLC
an Andrews McMeel Universal company
1130 Walnut Street, Kansas City, Missouri 64106

www.andrewsmcmeel.com

Produced by Authorscape, Inc.

12 13 14 15 16 RR3 10 9 8 7 6 5 4 3 2 1

ISBN: 978-1-4494-2761-0

Library of Congress Control Number: 2012938487

Secrets of Longevity® and Ask Dr. Mao® are registered trademarks of Ask Dr. Mao, LLC. Tao of Wellness® is a registered trademark of Tao of Wellness, PC.

For more information, go to www.askdrmao.com

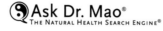

Ask Dr. Mao®
THE NATURAL HEALTH SEARCH ENGINE®

ATTENTION: SCHOOLS AND BUSINESSES

Andrews McMeel books are available at quantity discounts with bulk purchase for educational, business, or sales promotional use. For information, please e-mail the Andrews McMeel Publishing Special Sales Department: specialsales@amuniversal.com

NOTE TO THE READER:
This book is intended to provide helpful and informative material, and it is provided with the understanding that the author and publisher are not engaged in rendering medical, health, or any other kind of personal professional services in this compilation. Natural remedies and supplements can have side effects, both alone and in combination with other remedies or conventional medicines. The user of this book should consult his or her medical, health, or other competent professional before adopting any of the suggestions in this book or drawing inferences from them. The author and publisher specifically disclaim all responsibility for any liability, loss or risk, personal or otherwise, which is incurred as a consequence, directly or indirectly, of the use and application of any of the contents of this book.

Statements contained herein have not been evaluated by the U.S. Food and Drug Administration. The products referred to in this manual are not intended to diagnose, treat, cure, or prevent disease. Always consult with your professional healthcare and medical provider(s) before changing or discontinuing any medication.

To those interested in health, longevity, and good food—here's to your youthful vitality!

HEALTH KEY

The recipes in this book have been created to benefit your health in a variety of ways. Some may be good for your heart, while others promote healthy metabolism and digestion. As you go through the recipes, you'll notice that the benefits of each one are listed below the title. These ten categories and their benefits include:

1. HEART
Helpful for heart disease, high cholesterol, high blood pressure, pre-diabetes conditions, and diabetes.

2. IMMUNITY
Boosts immune system and supports cancer prevention.

3. ANTI-INFLAMMATION
Helpful for arthritis, muscle pain, and other inflammatory conditions.

4. METABOLISM
Increases energy, boosts metabolic function, and assists with weight loss.

5. CLEANSING
Supports the body in detoxification.

6. DIGESTION
Helpful for regularity, absorbing nutrients, and relieving heartburn, gas, and bloating.

7. BRAIN & VISION
Enhances cognitive function and eyesight.

8. ANTI-AGING BEAUTY
Benefits skin, hair, and nails.

9. GOOD MOOD
Restores happiness and alleviates stress.

10. SEXUAL HEALTH
Supports hormonal health and sexual health for women and men.

CONTENTS

LONGEVITY PRINCIPLES

Introduction 1

Thrive with Healing Foods .8

Kitchen Makeover 21

Eating and Cooking for Longevity 37

Spice for Life 47

Menus for Healing 50

RECIPES

Beverages 58

Breakfasts 72

Soups 86

Salads 104

Small Dishes 116

Snacks 158

Desserts 168

RESOURCES

References and Resources .174

Acknowledgments 179

Index 180

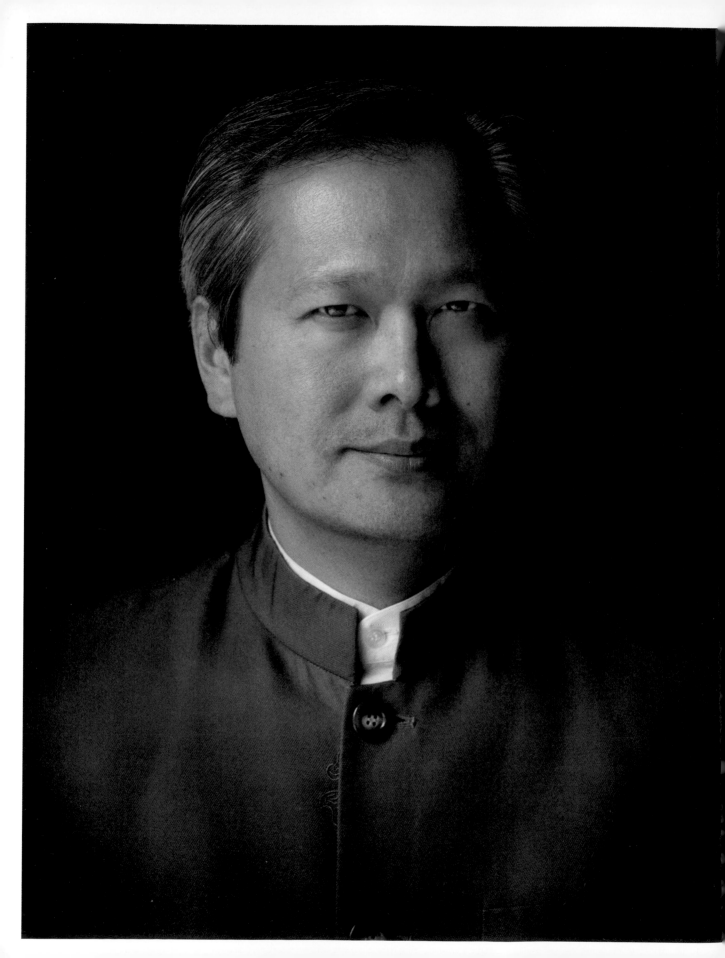

INTRODUCTION

"The doctor of the future will give no medication, but will interest his patients in the care of the human frame, diet, and in the cause and prevention of disease." —THOMAS A. EDISON

Today, many doctors and pharmaceutical companies would like you to believe that you need dose after dose of medical intervention and drugs to stay healthy and live longer. Centenarians—individuals who live to or beyond the age of 100 years—know this course of action is simply not beneficial. When asked, centenarians will tell you that the greatest secret to a long, fulfilling life is that *you* hold the key to your own longevity. You simply need to listen to your body and treat yourself with the respect and kindness you deserve! Your body was designed to last 100 years or more and as a result, you already possess the innate ability to heal yourself at every level—all you have to do is get out of your own way. Eating a healing diet of living, natural foods is your strongest ally in getting out of your own way and activating your own self-healing mechanisms. A balanced diet truly is the cornerstone to your longevity and healthy food is the greatest healer of all. It's time for us all to take the centenarians' wise advice: we need to take control of our own health, NOW!

I am passionate about the wisdom shared in this book and the powerful recipes that I have cherished and collected from long-living centenarians throughout my life and career. I know the secrets in this book can transform you in body, mind, and spirit—and support you in living a long, fulfilled life full of excellent health. Food is not the enemy. Food can be your greatest healer, and when its power is harnessed with knowledge, you can become your own greatest doctor. It is my hope that this cookbook will plant a small seed in changing the way you look at food, which in turn will inspire you to feed your body so you can thrive as centenarians have done for generations.

Eating to Thrive in the Modern Age: A Call to Action

Americans have a short memory when it comes to food. Not so long ago, we sourced all our food from neighboring farms and lovingly prepared wholesome and nutritious meals for ourselves and our families. Nowadays, most adults find themselves struggling to stay emotionally and physically healthy while managing busy careers, juggling families, and taking care of other responsibilities. Unfortunately, on the mental to-do list of the day, most adults place their personal health last. Instead of making time to shop for fresh produce, trying out new recipes, and spending time enjoying food with our community of family and friends, we oftentimes find ourselves racing out the door, grabbing a cup of coffee and a sugary snack, or bringing home take-out meals loaded with empty calories and very few nutrients. On any given day, we fall into bed and wonder to ourselves why we're often sick or why we always feel exhausted. We fail to make the true connection: we're not feeding ourselves well and our bodies are paying the price.

We often rush through each meal as if it were a chore, thinking of food merely as fast fuel, rarely enjoying the taste because we are always on the go. Furthermore, we are living at a time where it is easy to overeat, yet still be undernourished. Again and again, people eat high quantities of food with far too many empty calories and far too few nutrients. All of these factors are slowing down our metabolism and worsening our national health as rates of heart disease, cancer, and diabetes are all on the rise. The trusted so-called solutions—fad diets, prescriptions, expensive medical interventions that could be avoided—further add to the systemic problem, all while depleting our personal health, energy, and well-being. Taking all of this into account, it is easy to see that as a nation, we are gaining weight and taking years off our lives. This is a serious problem that we need to address NOW.

It is never too late to do an about-face and regain control of one's health! We have the ability to get back to eating real food that will help our health flourish. By committing to gradual and lasting change, we can slowly but surely heal ourselves and regain our instinctive nature to listen to our bodies, eat well, and enjoy life more. In many other parts of the world, eating is the focus of LIVING, a time for gathering with loved ones and enjoying a meal together. Food plays a key role in living *la dolce vita*—the sweet life. Isn't that the life we all dream of?

The longevity recipes in this cookbook come from a world of the past—a world before our modern agricultural system took control of farming techniques and food production methods, before corporate marketing executives and advertisers promoted addictive flavors and the glitzy, persuasive packaging of foods. But we cannot completely blame the modern world for our woeful state of health. The choice of what you feed yourself is yours alone. YOU get to decide whether to subsist on dead, lifeless foods or whether to choose living, breathing, healing foods.

Initially, you may cringe at the idea of giving up "convenience" foods, but I want you to consider this: is it really convenient to eat poor quality now, only to have to spend extra time and money at the doctor's office a few years later—not to mention the complete diminishment of your quality of life in the interim? It is an empowering enterprise to take back control over what you eat and how you feed your body. A healthy diet is the most powerful tool you have to feel energized, youthful, and on the path to true longevity.

The Longevity Cookbook Philosophy

My goal for this cookbook is to introduce you to a variety of healthy, tasty food from around the world. You will find recipes from many of the most famous "longevity capitals" of the world, including Okinawa, Japan; Vilcabamba, Ecuador; the Hunza Valley of Pakistan; Sardinia, Italy; and Bama County of China. The cookbook also features traditional recipes from Canada, Georgia, Poland, Russia, various Mediterranean countries, the Middle East, and Scandinavia. With easy-to-follow recipes for breakfasts, energy-boosting shakes, salads, soups, vegetarian dishes, meat dishes, snacks, and even desserts, there is something in this collection for everyone.

The simple philosophy of this cookbook is that by following the dietary wisdom of the centenarians, we can initiate self-healing within ourselves, enjoy life more in the present, and achieve longevity in the future. There are eight key components to this philosophy, which are woven throughout this book.

1. EAT FIVE SMALLER MEALS A DAY

The recipes in this cookbook are smaller in size than what we are traditionally accustomed to in the U.S. My inspiration came from Spanish *tapas*, the delightful snack-sized dishes that allow you to eat slowly and savor the food's flavor while enjoying conversation with family and friends. The recipes in this book offer a wide variety of snack-sized items from around the world, which are easy to prepare, tasty for children and adults alike, and are supportive to your health and longevity. While the recommended portion sizes of meals are smaller, the number of total meals per day is greater. I believe you should eat five *tapas*-sized meals a day to distribute an even stream of energy and nutrients to your body throughout the day.

2. COMBINE THE BEST OF THE EAST AND WEST

These longevity recipes integrate many ancient healing traditions of the East as well as simple time-saving tricks of the West. When you make these recipes, you will benefit from thousands of years of Eastern observation and experience, coupled with modern Western research and science. Implementing these two complementary approaches of traditional wisdom with modern advances will provide you with the very best techniques of eating to truly THRIVE.

3. CONSUME MORE PLANTS

I am a firm believer that a plant-based diet is paramount for achieving longevity. If you look at the famous longevity capitals of the world—such as Okinawa, Vilcabamba, Hunza Valley, Sardinia, Georgia, and Bama—what the inhabitants naturally eat in all those locations are plenty of fresh vegetables, protein-rich beans, sometimes fish, and very little meat or modern processed foods. These cultures traditionally emphasize eating plants and natural foods, and as a result, they have much lower rates of the top diseases facing modern society, including heart disease, cancer, liver disease, and degenerative diseases.

Western science has confirmed the lasting health benefits of a diet high in vegetables and fish and low in animal products. The famous China Study, a large-scale, twenty-year study of 6,500 people in China, written by T. Colin Campbell, Ph.D. and Thomas M. Campbell, demonstrated the huge impact that a low-fat, high-fiber diet has on maintaining good health and avoiding chronic diseases now associated with a Westernized diet. The Chinese countryside dwellers featured in the study had a diet that was at least 80 percent plant foods, while only roughly 7 percent of their total protein came from animal products—and they had low rates of heart disease, colon cancer, and osteoporosis. Sadly, it can be noted that when the rural dweller moved to the city and adopted the urban lifestyle and diet of higher fat, more heavily processed foods, diseases increased.

4. EAT HEALING FOODS AND AVOID RAPID-AGING FOODS

The key players in these longevity recipes are nutritious, plant-based foods with extraordinary healing powers: vegetables, fruits, grains, beans, legumes, seaweeds, nuts, and seeds, with fish and/or poultry playing a supporting role. You will notice that just about every recipe in this book is low-sodium, sugar-free, gluten-free, and dairy-free. The health benefits of avoiding these substances are well-documented, and you can learn all about these life-shortening culprits in the section "Thrive with Healing Foods." This section will also give you advice on navigating our Western food system to make the best food choices for your health, safety, and longevity.

Keep in mind that the majority of the previously mentioned diseases are preventable—YOU have the power to regain your longevity and say no to high-fat, processed foods. Eating these rapid-aging foods is depriving many people of their natural lifespan, and many more of their zest for life, which is a needless shame. The proven health benefits of eating a plant-based diet are life-giving. When the diet is also dairy-free, sugar-free, and gluten-free, the benefits are astounding! You will be amazed at the results stemming from this life-changing diet.

5. PREPARE YOUR KITCHEN FOR LONGEVITY

You can only eat as well as your pantry is stocked and your kitchen is equipped. If your cupboard is bare—or worse, filled with sugary treats that pack on the pounds and shorten your years—you will greatly benefit from the section "Kitchen Makeover," which gives simple tips for stocking the pantry. You may be surprised to learn that there are potentially nutrient-destroying foods and life-shortening toxins lurking in your kitchen and you will also want to make over your cooking equipment to best support your longevity.

6. EAT AND COOK LIKE A CENTENARIAN

This cookbook is about not only what foods to eat for longevity, but also how best to prepare them, when to eat, how much to eat, and where—or where not!—to eat. In the section "Eating and Cooking for Longevity" you will learn the ten golden rules that centenarians follow to preserve health and prolong life.

7. LET FOOD BE YOUR MEDICINE

A very useful section, "Menus for Healing" outlines supportive menus for specific health conditions—including weight loss, heart health, immunity, and inflammatory conditions. The menus are based on the smaller five-meal approach and the recipes help guide you through what you can eat for five meals a day, seven days a week.

8. ENJOY THE SWEET LIFE

Most importantly, this book is about relishing the food you eat and enjoying the process of making it. Despite the best intentions, many "healthy" cookbooks offer recipes that can be on the bland side, leading to the common complaint that health food is boring, flavorless, or downright distasteful. The healthy recipes in this book are bold, flavorful, and filled with the exciting variety that comes from various cooking traditions. That's why I call this centenarian-based cooking approach eating to thrive—not eating to deprive! Cooking is an adventure, and no more so than when you are preparing a new recipe with your family or trying a new cooking technique in your kitchen. *La dolce vita* should be enjoyed and savored!

BE SAFE

Keep in mind that food-drug interaction can sometimes occur, meaning that the food you eat can inhibit medicine from working the way it should. For instance, grapefruit counteracts the cholesterol-lowering properties of statin drugs; leafy greens containing vitamin K can potentially hinder effectiveness of blood thinners like Coumadin; citrus juices may decrease the efficacy of certain antibiotics. As your health strategies change and evolve, remember to never stop taking prescription medications without first speaking to your physician about your dietary goals and plans. A smart approach to longevity includes balancing all aspects of one's health: food, necessary medication(s), exercise, and emotional well-being.

The Origin of Longevity Recipes

I want to conclude with what most inspired me to put this book together: the truly remarkable longevity recipes I received from the dynamic centenarians I count myself lucky to have met. From 1985 to 2005, I extensively interviewed over a hundred centenarians in China, with a special interest in observing what foods they ate and recipes they shared with their families. Many of this book's recipes are taken from the life-changing lessons they shared with me.

In addition to centenarian interviews, several of these recipes come from my generous patients, students, and friends I have met over the course of my career. My patients at the Tao of Wellness in Los Angeles and students from Yo San University come from all over the world and all walks of life. At the Tao of Wellness, my colleagues and I perform roughly 50,000 treatments every year—so that should give you some idea that these recipes truly come from a very wide and diverse spectrum! During my initial session with a new patient, I always begin with a discussion to assess every aspect of their health. When a patient is in very good health at an advanced age, I immediately ask them, "What is your favorite thing to eat?" and scribble down the foods and recipes as quickly as I can.

Younger patients sometimes mention a particularly long-lived family member, and I find out what they liked to eat the most. What's so unique about many of these recipes is that they are passed down through families and generations, like a priceless heirloom or jewel. I am blessed to have such generous patients who are willing to share their family recipes with me and it is my hope that these recipes may now become part of your family's traditions to be treasured and passed down to future generations.

Finally, a few of these recipes are cooking techniques I grew up with in my youth. They reflect my family's thirty-eight generations of traditional Chinese medicine—and my mother's own innovative ways to keep two hungry boys happy! I feel blessed to have grown up surrounded by such healing wisdom at my own dinner table.

I was sparked to action to create this book by the centenarians I met and learned from, and I hope you, too, are inspired by them to cook these simple, wholesome recipes with the intention of eating to thrive. I challenge you to follow the advice in this book for at least a full week, and see if you don't feel more vital, energized, and healthy. Give it a try—you will inspire yourself.

You are what you eat, so eat like a centenarian and embrace your longevity!

THRIVE WITH HEALING FOODS

"Let food be thy medicine, and medicine be thy food." —HIPPOCRATES

Hippocrates perfectly sums up the healing power of food in the statement above. Diet and nutrition are powerful healers in traditional Chinese medicine and in many other Eastern traditions. The new science of functional foods studies the healing and regenerative power of whole foods, which contain powerful compounds and antioxidants that help prevent disease and improve organ function. I strongly believe that if we commit to eating healthy, natural foods, we can positively *thrive* with health and longevity!

This informative section celebrates the healing and life-saving superfoods and unmasks various food villains that are rapidly shortening your life. A Catalan proverb states, "From the bitterness of disease man learns the sweetness of health." It is my sincere hope that we can avoid the bitterness of disease—and instead enjoy the sweetness of good health by changing the way we eat and choosing superfoods to thrive.

Healing, Anti-Aging Foods

For thousands of years, humans treated their bodies as personal laboratories to discover which foods were therapeutic and which were poisonous. Prehistoric humans evaluated "healthy" and "unhealthy" foods based on their reactions to what they put in their mouths. Occasionally, eating a certain food, herb, or plant would bring relief to a particular ailment, and that food would be noted as possessing healing qualities. Over time, patterns emerged and were combined into longstanding principles governing healthy diet and nutrition. After thousands of years of experimentation and documentation, and with the consensus of modern science, it is widely agreed that fresh fruits and vegetables should be humans' primary foods. Fruits and vegetables are low in fat and sodium, high in fiber, and best of all, these superfoods are packed with powerful antioxidants crucial for maintaining your health.

All whole, unprocessed foods from the earth—fruits, vegetables, grains, beans and legumes, nuts, and seeds—possess rich, healing properties. Take just one example: cranberries. Cranberries are antioxidant-rich and have been traditionally used in the prevention and treatment of urinary tract issues. While perceptive and health-conscious humans have recognized this truth for centuries, studies now show that cranberries contain hippuric acid, which inhibits the growth and attachment of various strains of bacteria, such as E. coli, to the bladder. Studies also prove that cranberries improve dental health and help heal stomach ulcers by inhibiting *H. pylori*. Cranberries are merely one healing food in your arsenal to achieve good health and longevity!

Top Ten Healing, Anti-Aging Foods

In my twenty-year studies of centenarians, I discovered that the same ten foods kept recurring again and again in the diets of long-living individuals. There are plenty of wonderful healing foods, but I believe these to be the best when it comes to longevity and self-healing:

1. Sweet potatoes
2. Corn
3. Peanuts
4. Pumpkin
5. Walnuts
6. Black beans
7. Sesame seeds
8. Shiitake mushrooms
9. Green tea
10. Seaweed

Rapid-Aging Foods

Now that we have a short list of healing superfoods, you may be wondering about the foods that are causing us the most harm. These foods include sugar, sodium, dairy, gluten, caffeine, alcohol, and fatty foods, as well as processed and pre-packaged convenience foods.

The centenarians I have come to know almost entirely avoid these foods, which accounts for much of their health and vitality. These foods have very little nutrient power or health benefits to offer, except for an intensely unnatural flavor that we have been sold on and have grown accustomed to craving. But there is a reason these foods are called "junk" food! They are a poor-quality fuel: high in calories, but low in nutrition. Would you put gasoline into your car that caused it to frequently break down? You should think of your body in the same way. Over time, poor-quality fuel will cease to sustain the proper function of your body, and you will have continual breakdowns in health. When you're sustaining yourself on 1,500 to 2,000 calories every day, you want to make sure every calorie counts with nutrient-rich and antioxidant-packed foods!

For those of you who mourn the idea of giving up sugary, salty snacks, take heart! It is a common misconception that healthy foods lack flavor. Indeed, unprocessed foods offer many more complex and delightful flavors than a bag of salty chips or package of sugary cookies. Imagine the aroma and taste of a fresh tomato, a bunch of garden-grown basil, or the sweet juiciness of a perfectly ripe peach. Our taste buds have grown accustomed to tastes created by chemists in food labs, designed to make us eat past our point of fullness in order to make us eat more and therefore buy more. Sadly, our health has been swapped in exchange for the profits of moneymaking businesses.

This book is not meant to scare or dishearten you into giving up all your favorite foods overnight, or into tossing out all of your favorite recipes! Start slowly to gradually cut back on processed foods and to incorporate more whole foods into your diet. As you gently ease yourself through this transition, your taste buds will adjust and become more finely tuned to taste far more exciting flavors than just sugar and salt. Most importantly, I am a firm believer that moderation is the healthiest path. A glass of wine or a cookie once in a while isn't going to kill you—these treats should simply be enjoyed in moderation.

REFINED SUGAR: DON'T BE TRICKED BY TREATS

The science surrounding sugar is very clear. Eating too much refined sugar can lead to diabetes, heart disease, inflammation, cancer, obesity, and other diseases that will diminish your quality of life and will certainly lessen your years. Most people are aware of this truth, and yet the average American today consumes between 140 and 200 pounds of sugar per year. Meanwhile, in the 1800's, the average American consumed 20 pounds or less of sugar per year. A century ago in the United States, there were far fewer cases of diabetes, compared with today's approximately 8.3 percent incidence of diabetes. Such a drastic change makes you think—we need to change our poor eating habits and get back on track with healthy, balanced food!

Sugar doesn't just affect your long-term health. Too much sugar can also immediately affect your immune system and mood, perhaps giving you an initial lift, but often leaving you depressed, anxious, sluggish, or otherwise not functioning at full capacity. One study found that when subjects were given refined sugar, their white blood cell count decreased significantly for several hours afterwards—which is terrible news for your immune system. More research is needed, but sugar is also being implicated in certain behavioral disorders.

Using the previously mentioned statistics, the average American is eating nearly half a pound of sugar per *day*! How is that possible? One main reason is that refined sugar is in just about everything found in the grocery store: pre-packaged cakes, cookies, candy, jelly, bread, sauces and condiments, and even salty snacks. Most of this excess sugar ends up being stored as fat in our bodies, resulting in weight gain and elevating risks of heart disease and cancer. Sugar also increases blood pressure, especially in people who are overweight. So cut out the sugar and seek sweetness from your life instead!

Swap for: Honey, maple syrup, stevia, fresh fruits and berries—in moderation! See more specific options in the "Pantry Essentials" section, starting on page 21.

SALT: PASS ON IT

It should come as no surprise that most of us use *far* too much salt! A little salt is generally all right, and in fact, salt is important for certain bodily functions, but excessive salt intake leads to heart disease, causes elevation of blood pressure, creates water retention, and may increase risks of osteoporosis. Additionally, recent studies have shown that increased salt intake is proportional to an increase in cancers of the stomach, esophagus, and bladder. In comparison, populations that consume low amounts of salt do not experience blood pressure rates as high as those seen in most Western countries.

The average American consumes nearly two teaspoons of sodium (between 3,400 and 3,700 milligrams) a day, far exceeding the national dietary recommendation of no more than 2,300 milligrams, or one teaspoon a day, and 1,500 milligrams for those who have or are at risk for high blood pressure. You may think the salt shaker is to blame, but actually, the majority of the salt we consume is hidden in packaged, processed foods as well as in restaurant meals, including fast food. Fear not, there are far more varied flavors that will create dishes so tasty that you won't even miss the added salt.

Swap for: Herbs, spices, vinegars, or a squeeze of fresh lemon. See more specific options in the "Pantry Essentials" section, starting on page 21.

DAIRY: STICK TO ORGANIC, HORMONE-FREE PRODUCTS

It's a common misconception that dairy is the only good source of calcium in everyday foods—in fact, it is one of the more difficult calcium sources for the human body to process. Most people around the world actually don't get their daily intake of calcium from dairy. (A significant number of people are lactose-intolerant and also, it's simply not viable to use large portions of land solely for dairy cows in many regions.) The majority of people around the world obtain their calcium from beans, legumes, and leafy green vegetables, from which the body is much more easily able to access calcium-rich nutrients.

In particular, processed dairy products in the U.S. lack a great deal of nutrients and vitamins. Due to the high volume of dairy products required to feed roughly 300 million people, U.S. regulations impose tight restrictions on dairy farms and processing plants, requiring pasteurization and homogenization techniques. While these regulations are in place for our safety, the processes often strip commercial dairy products of their flavor and much of their nutrients. Furthermore, most U.S. dairies over-medicate livestock with large amounts of antibiotics and most farms lack the acreage needed to let livestock graze on grass. As a result, most livestock are fed a diet of processed corn products and grain. To boost milk production, livestock are also given body-altering hormones. Not only do such living conditions and treatments negatively affect the milk that is processed and sold in the U.S., but our soil and water supply are also negatively affected. My personal feeling is that you want all of your food—including dairy products—to be as natural and close to the source as possible, with minimal processing.

Dairy products are produced very differently in other parts of the world. European dairy farmers produce their milk on a much smaller scale and as a result, most livestock are grass-fed rather than grain-fed, so the farmers can better control safety and preserve the milk's nutrients without using pasteurization or antibiotics. These measures, in turn, result in far fewer allergies to milk and less disruption to the digestive system than in the U.S. Additionally, the flavor of milk is delightfully varied and preserved in Europe, based on the different animals, location, climate, and grass type. In the U.S., we impose that every commercially sold jug of milk taste exactly the same, and in keeping with this method, large-scale farms produce milk in the same way.

If you are going to eat dairy products, it is my recommendation that you join a community dairy co-operative so as to purchase products from a nearby dairy farmer who operates the farm on a small scale without antibiotics or pesticides. Most importantly, you should commit to buying only organic, hormone-free dairy products.

Also, I make some exception for yogurt and kefir because it is fermented food, which helps restore flora. I prefer products made from milk other than cow's milk because lactose is often difficult to digest, so I generally recommend sheep's milk yogurt, goat's milk yogurt, soy yogurt, rice yogurt, and coconut yogurt, all of which are available at health-food stores.

Swap for: Plant milk, especially almond, hemp, or soy. See more specific options in the "Pantry Essentials" section, starting on page 21.

GLUTEN: DIFFICULT TO DIGEST

Gluten is a composite formed from several different proteins that are found primarily in wheat and related grains, like rye and barley. Gluten can be difficult for the body to process and digest, and many people develop a sensitivity to it. Many individuals suffer from celiac disease and cannot process gluten at all. Over the past several decades, celiac disease and gluten intolerance have become increasingly prevalent in modern, developed countries. I believe that much of the problem lies with the manner in which wheat and other gluten grains are now commercially produced on a very large scale, including the widespread use of genetic engineering to produce new traits in wheat. Why create wheat hybrids and make genetic changes in the first place? One motivation is to create a wheat strain that is better equipped to withstand harsh weather or insects, while another reason is to produce a wheat strain that works well in the making of bread or pasta. The genetic engineering of wheat and other grains has resulted in crops that are no longer classifiable as plants, but are rather labelled genetically modified organisms (GMOs). Some believe that the widespread genetic engineering and hybridization of wheat has resulted in a huge increase of the gluten content of today's wheat, in comparison to the untampered-with wheat of a century ago. It's no wonder celiac disease and gluten intolerance have increased so alarmingly in the last thirty years!

At the Tao of Wellness, we find that by removing gluten from our patients' diets, most patients feel better mentally and physically. I believe gluten reduction also leads to lower stress and more balanced emotional levels, both of which make a lasting difference in how people feel. If you decide to cut out gluten products completely, take care to make sure you are still eating a balanced diet and incorporating other low-sugar carbohydrates.

Swap for: Wheatless grains and flours. See more specific options in the "Pantry Essentials" section, starting on page 21.

COFFEE: SWITCH TO TEA

Some studies have shown that coffee may help lower the risk of diabetes and help you live slightly longer. Obviously the reported benefits of coffee are negated once it's doctored with high-fat cream, sugary syrup, or processed sweeteners. Additionally those with high blood pressure, anxiety, and insomnia should avoid coffee.

If you want to drink a healthier beverage that will help energize you, drink the beverage of centenarians: tea. High in antioxidants and polyphenols, tea lowers rates of heart disease and cancer. Whereas coffee hot-wires your nerves and depletes your life force in the long run, tea gently lifts your energy. Black, green, white, and oolong teas all contain antioxidant polyphenols, with green and white tea taking the lead for the highest amounts. In fact, tea ranks as high as or higher than many fruits and vegetables in the Oxygen Radical Absorbance Capacity (ORAC) scale, a score that measures antioxidant potential of plant-based foods. Herbal tea does not have the same antioxidant properties, though it is still delicious and beneficial for other healthy effects, such as inducing relaxation and relieving stress.

Swap for: Green, white, or herbal tea.

ALCOHOL: RISKY BUSINESS

Alcohol is highly destructive to your body, particularly your liver. The liver is one of the hardest-working organs in your body and performs a wide variety of functions. Its most important functions include processing nutrients, producing bile to help with food digestion and waste elimination, and cleansing the blood of toxins such as alcohol and other dangerous substances. The liver has the ability to regenerate itself, but the adverse effects of alcohol eventually wear it down.

Several studies have found that drinking excessive amounts of alcohol can raise blood pressure to unhealthy levels. But, wait, you may ask, what about the French tradition of drinking wine daily? It is true that consuming red wine correlates to a lower risk of heart disease—however, the French have a higher incidence of cirrhosis of the liver. In this scenario, you are trading heart disease for liver problems. Too much alcohol has also been linked to cancer. Women especially should take note that alcohol increases the risk of breast cancer. Keep in mind that alcohol is high in calories and can also contribute to unwanted weight gain.

Should you cut out alcohol forever? As you've already learned, a healthy diet is about balance and moderation—a small glass of wine with dinner a couple times a week is perfectly fine. Stick to this rule of thumb: limit drinking to the weekend, and have no more than one glass each day. Also, listen to your body's personal tolerance level. If you can't tolerate alcohol, don't violate your body.

Swap for: Nonalcoholic drinks, like unsweetened iced tea or water with a twist of lemon.

MEAT: MAKE SMART CHOICES

I believe that Americans should stop thinking of meat as the sole centerpiece of the meal. This is not to say that you shouldn't eat meat at all, but rather that meat doesn't need to be in the oversize portions that we have come to expect, and it does not need to be in every meal we consume. Try eating meat only three or four days a week, in 4- to 5-ounce portions—approximately the size of a deck of cards. Choose free-range, grass-fed, and hormone- and antibiotic-free meat, which is much healthier for both you and the planet. You will see in these recipes that when I cook with meat, I almost always use fish and poultry, mostly steering away from fatty red meat.

Swap for: Grains and beans, combined with delicious veggies to fill out your meal.

TO SUPPLEMENT OR NOT TO SUPPLEMENT?

I believe you should get your daily nutrients out of food as much as possible, and you can do this by eating plenty of vegetables, fruits, grains, beans and legumes, nuts and seeds, healthy meats, and seaweeds. That said, there are cases in which it makes sense to supplement your diet with vitamins. Vegetarians should take vitamin B_{12} and possibly vitamin D, since they are missing out on these nutrients by not eating meat. Pregnant women should take extra folic acid. Those with osteoporosis will need to take extra calcium, magnesium, trace minerals like boron, and other supplements that specifically support their bone health. People recovering from a long illness may need to take certain immune-boosting supplements.

It's important to keep in mind that the American soil from which most of our food derives from is significantly depleted of nutrients, and as a result, our food isn't as nutritious as it once was, which begs the question of whether we are even getting enough nutrients by eating a wide variety of foods. If this is of concern to you, you may consider taking a general mineral supplement or daily multivitamin. Whenever possible, ingest supplements that are extracted from whole foods like fruits, vegetables, and grains. These will have the best bioavailability, meaning the highest absorption rate by your digestive system. The best way to take vitamins and minerals is in powdered form, liquid concentrate, or as oil. Avoid taking mega-doses or any dose larger than the recommended dietary reference intakes, no matter how good they may be for your health.

Supplementing your diet with vitamins should be the exception, not the rule; they are, after all, called supplements. Nutrients are much more accessible and easily processed by your body when they are consumed in food form versus supplement form. Also, there is the danger that a person taking vitamins will then rationalize that there is no need to focus on balanced nutrition from food—but there is no magic bullet and no replacement for a diet of healthy, whole foods.

Get to Know Your Food

Shopping for longevity starts with knowing where your food comes from and what it specifically contains. The only way to protect your health and preserve your longevity in the confusing marketplace is to do your due diligence: research where your food is coming from, how it is produced, and how it is transported. Have a chat with the fishmonger or the attendant at the farmer's stand; you'll learn a wealth of information about your food!

You have the most control of what you feed your body by cooking wholesome, nutritious recipes from scratch in your own kitchen. Of course, this practice is ideal, but sometimes you will find yourself in a restaurant or at a friend's home for dinner. If you are constantly agonizing over how the food was produced or sourced, you will drive yourself crazy and upset your digestion. Control what you can control by preparing the majority of your meals at home. The rest of the time, just relax and enjoy the company of good friends and family!

CHOOSE LOCAL, IN-SEASON FOODS

Your diet should follow the seasons, and you should primarily eat what grows locally. Nature has the perfect plan for providing you with the appropriate foods for each season. The fruits and vegetables that ripen in the summer, including watermelon, collard greens, and zucchini, tend to be on the cooling side to counter the heat of the season. Winter's variety of produce offers warming foods, including leeks, onions, and turnips. When you shop primarily at your local farmer's market instead of a large grocery chain store, you will begin to get a better sense of what is in season at different times of the year, and by doing so, you will feed your body what it needs most.

Fresh, local produce contains more nutrients than refrigerated and/or canned fruits and vegetables. Furthermore, local produce is picked when it is naturally ripe. On the other hand, commercial produce transported from other countries is picked unripe and treated with chemicals to ripen artificially late. Produce is then shipped hundreds or even thousands of miles on a week-long, sometimes even month-long, trip before it is served on your dining table—negatively affecting your stomach and also the planet. Each step in the long process minimizes the nutrients and flavor of your food even more. So, in short, eat fresh food grown close to home. It's better for your health, better for the environment, and has an unbeatable taste. That's what I call win-win-win!

GO ORGANIC FOR NUTRIENTS AND SAFETY

One of the most often heard complaints about organic foods is that they are so much more expensive than commercially grown produce. People often ask, is it really worth the extra money? For one thing, what you may save in money now on commercial produce, you are surely losing in health later if you get sick after eating chemically-treated fruit and vegetables. Eating as much organic produce as possible will help protect you from ingesting the toxins and chemicals that are very quickly becoming widespread in our food supply. Many scientific studies have shown that organic foods have a much higher percentage of antioxidants than non-organic foods. Other studies continue to emerge about the negative effects of pesticides and herbicides used on commercial crops, including increased cancer risk, inflammation, hormonal imbalances, and reproductive issues in humans and animals.

If you want the health benefits of eating organic without sacrificing your entire budget, focus on purchasing key organic foods that matter most. The twelve fruits and vegetables that are frequently found to be high in pesticide levels are apples, celery, strawberries, peaches, spinach, nectarines (imported), grapes (imported), sweet bell peppers, potatoes, blueberries (domestic), lettuce, and kale or collard greens. By buying local, organic versions of these foods, you can reduce your pesticide exposure by almost 80 percent!

When tested, these conventionally grown commercial foods have the least amount of pesticides: avocados, asparagus, broccoli, cabbage, eggplant, kiwi, mangos, onions, papaya, pineapples, sweet corn, sweet peas, sweet potatoes, tomatoes, and watermelon.

You should also know that even some organic foods aren't completely immune from the dangers of modern-day food production methods, but they offer your best chance to eat nutrient-rich food safely, without that food being covered in dangerous chemicals. Whether you go for conventional or organic, make sure to always wash all of your produce thoroughly before eating.

While the main focus of this section is produce, eggs and meat should also be organic and sourced as locally as possible for freshness. If you can, purchase your animal products at an organic butcher or from a local farmer who knows the background of his or her products. Try to make sure the meat is grass-fed and free of antibiotics, hormones, and other chemicals. It's also good practice to ask your butcher to remove excess fat from meat and poultry, as this is where most of the toxins in the animal are stored.

Farmer's markets and health-food stores are increasingly found nationwide. Even large grocery store chains carry organic foods, so no matter where you shop, you should be able to find nutritious, safe foods to grace your dinner table.

AVOID GMO FOODS

It's important to avoid foods that contain genetically modified organisms (GMOs) because they have been manipulated in a lab to make a plant more productive, more resistant to pests, or to contain higher amounts of a certain nutrient. When plants are made to be more productive, it is really no different than using growth hormones in animals or athletes taking steroids. These practices promote extremely rapid growth in the short term but have negative side effects down the road. It will take several generations to see how the human body adapts to genetically engineered foods, and what the serious, long-term, and harmful side effects will be.

We are oftentimes slow to change our habits in the U.S., waiting until the last possible moment—which can sometimes be too late—to implement a positive solution. Europe has always led the way with its approach to banning environmental toxins, pesticides, hormones, and GMOs. Until our nation begins to widely recognize these hazards, we can take a cue from Europe, at least on an individual basis. If a product is outlawed in Europe, then outlaw it for yourself. Read up on the research, stay informed, and make adjustments in your diet as new material surfaces.

FISH SAFETY

As more people discover the healthy, tasty benefits of fresh fish, they also find that there are many confusing issues related to toxins and problems associated with overfishing.

The rule of thumb for toxins in fish is: larger and older fish tend to have the highest levels of mercury. Mercury is a naturally occurring metal and is increasingly found in our food sources and environment. When it is combined with other elements, it forms inorganic mercury compounds. Mercury also combines with carbon to make a common compound called methylmercury, which is produced mainly by microscopic organisms in soil or water. This methylmercury, which may be formed in water, accumulates in the tissues of fish. Refrain from eating seafood that tends to have high levels of mercury, such as tuna, swordfish, tilefish, king mackerel, and shark. Most shellfish also contains traces of mercury, so limit your intake. Toxins are particularly dangerous for pregnant women, children, and infants. Do careful research to help you make appropriate choices.

Overfishing is a complicated problem with no easy answers. Your best bet is to make friends with a reputable fishmonger who will be more up-to-date on the shortages and dangers in your region's seafood.

BE A LABEL SLEUTH

This section emphasizes knowing more about the origin and production of your whole foods: produce, beans and legumes, and meats—and this is mainly because I recommend eating foods in their wholeness, where *you* are in control of how they are processed into a meal, rather than a company being in control of the processing. That being said, make sure you know exactly what is in packaged food, too. Don't be fooled by the bright and shiny claims on the front of the box—the real proof is on the nutrition facts and ingredients list. Look closely at the small print: if the ingredient list reminds you of Frankenstein's science lab and contains words you can't pronounce, stay away! Pay attention to the sodium, fiber, and fat content per serving size, and make sure the serving size is realistic. Check the expiration date. If the expiration date is several months or even years from the purchase date, you can be sure it's full of preservatives and has nothing nutritious to offer.

And of course, steer clear of all highly processed and refined foods that line grocery store shelves. As previously mentioned, these foods are stripped of critical nutrients and are full of unnecessary sugar, sodium, and other unnatural additives. Choose living foods now and eat them in their wholeness—without processing—whenever possible!

Red Flags in the Ingredient List

Packaged foods are full of nasty additives used to increase flavor and extend shelf life. These unnatural additives may extend the life of the food, but they will subtract years from yours. Choose foods in their wholeness whenever possible, but if you plan on buying any packaged food, make sure you avoid these:

- **Sodium chloride**—a little salt goes a long way. Too much salt can lead to high blood pressure, compromised cardiovascular health, and kidney failure. Sodium content shouldn't exceed 5 percent of the recommended daily intake.
- **Sugar** is an addictive substance with little nutritional value that can lead to weight gain, obesity, and diabetes. Watch out for these processed sugary components: high fructose corn syrup, glucose, confectioner's sugar, dextrose, maltose, fruit juice concentrate, powdered sugar, sucrose, invert sugar, corn sweetener, corn syrup.
- **Artificial sweeteners** are found in most "sugar-free" diet drinks, gums, candy bars, gelatins, and low-calorie desserts, usually in the form of Equal, Sweet 'N Low, Splenda, or other artificial sweeteners, most of which contain asparatame, sucralose, acesulfame K, and have been linked to cancer.
- **Trans fats** are used frequently in packaged foods to preserve freshness and extend the expiration date. These trans fats elevate your "bad" LDL cholesterol and make your "good" HDL plummet.
- **Monosodium glutamate (MSG)** is often added to salad dressings, canned goods, sauces, soups, chips, and many other processed foods. MSG has been linked to headaches, rapid heartbeat, nausea, chest pain, and overall body weakness.
- **Sodium nitrite** is often found in lunch meats, hot dogs, bacon, and smoked foods and has been linked to various types of cancer.
- **BHA** and **BHT** are often added to breakfast cereals, rice, chips, and other packaged foods to prevent the fats from going rancid. Although you would need to consume 125 times the amount added to foods to experience the full negative effects, there is still concern regarding their safety.
- **Olestra,** used in fat-free snacks, is a chemically produced, synthetic fat with reported side effects that include anal leakage, gas, and cramps.
- **Food colorings** are often made with petroleum and have been linked to cancer. Especially avoid Blue 1 and 2, Red 3, Green 3, and Yellow 6, which can show up in everything from candy to beverages to sausage.
- **Potassium bromate,** a carcinogenic used as a chemical leavening agent in flour, bread, and rolls, has been banned in Europe.

KITCHEN MAKEOVER

"Food is an implement of magic, and only the most coldhearted rationalist could squeeze the juices of life out of it and make it bland. In a true sense, a cookbook is the best source of psychological advice and the kitchen the first choice of room for a therapy of the world."

—SIR THOMAS MORE

Eating for health and longevity begins right in your own kitchen. Eating to thrive and cooking for longevity will most likely require you to make some changes in your kitchen, from the utensils you cook with to the visual cues you give yourself every time you walk in there. Take a look at your kitchen countertop and table. A bowl of fresh fruit in your line of vision is more likely to result in your eating an apple the next time you are hungry. A bag of chips, however, will probably lead to unhealthy choices. Part of your kitchen makeover includes making sure that your pantry is well stocked to support your longevity goals. Does this process mean you should throw out every bag of white rice and pasta you own? No, this transition is a gradual process that will continue to evolve as you make better choices about the food you eat and the way you prepare meals.

Stocking your kitchen with healthy tools is just as important as stocking your kitchen with healthy food. Open your cupboards and take a look at the pots, storage containers, and utensils. This may be the first time you ever gave serious thought to what tools are in your kitchen, but you should know that some popular Western cooking techniques, such as heating disposable plastic containers in the microwave and frequently using handy nonstick pans, may increase the levels of toxic chemicals in your food. Rest assured, the second half of this section is devoted to helping you pick the best kitchen tools for living a long, healthy life.

Pantry Essentials and Storage Tips

Closely examine your pantry and start tossing unhealthy or expired food while stocking up sensibly on healthier options. The exciting thing about restocking your pantry is that it is a process that will never be complete. Each week you can choose new, fresh items that will temporarily live there. Essentially, your pantry should be filled with subletting tenants, as opposed to long-term residents. Personally, I am against stocking up in bulk because most foods I recommend eating for longevity will spoil within a few months. In fact, the mark of a living food is that it will not last long when left sitting in your fridge or pantry. Choose the best-quality, organic, GMO-free foods for your health and safety.

FRUITS AND VEGGIES

All fresh fruits and vegetables are superfoods when it comes to health and longevity! Keep in mind that organic foods don't last as long as pesticide-treated foods, and quicker spoilage is to be expected. Buy just enough fresh organic produce to last you and your family a few days. There is no easy rule of thumb for preserving produce. Some produce does better in the refrigerator, some in a dark place in your pantry, and some best out on the counter to ripen for a day or two. I will say that your kitchen and your health will both benefit from a bowl of fresh fruit, including oranges, apples, bananas, kiwi fruit, limes, and lemons, in plain sight on your kitchen counter.

NUTS AND SEEDS

Most nuts and seeds will begin to spoil if kept more than two months. Interestingly, it is their healthy unsaturated fats that cause them to spoil relatively quickly. Unsaturated fats turn rancid more readily than saturated fats because their molecular structure leaves them more prone to oxidative damage. Nuts and seeds will last the longest if you put them in airtight containers, keep them in a dark spot, and refrigerate or freeze them. Nuts and seeds should also be bought as fresh as possible, preferably in their shells to be cracked open for eating. Below is a list of the nuts and seeds that show up frequently in this cookbook's longevity recipes.

- Almonds
- Black sesame seeds
- Chestnuts
- Dried whole chestnuts
- Flaxseeds
- Pecans

- Sunflower seeds
- Sesame seeds
- Peanuts
- Pine nuts
- Pumpkin seeds
- Walnuts

DRIED BEANS AND LEGUMES

If stored in airtight glass containers that are not exposed to sunlight, beans and legumes should last roughly six months in your pantry. Below is a list of the most nutrient-rich beans and legumes.

- Adzuki beans
- Black beans
- Black-eyed-peas
- Garbanzo beans
- Green lentils
- Green split peas
- Lima beans
- Kidney beans

- Mung beans
- Pink beans
- Pinto beans
- Red lentils
- Soybeans
- White beans
- Yellow split peas

No Can Do

I don't recommend buying canned foods because they are often packed with far too much sodium, and the cans can be lined with a hazardous compound known as bisphenol A (BPA), which may increase the risk of cancer and disrupt the endocrine system. I recommend buying your beans, fish, and other foods fresh, but if you are very busy and it comes down to canned black beans or no black beans, go with the can. However, make sure the can was made in the U.S., there is no bump in the can or soldering line around the edge of the lid, which could indicate that lead was used to seal the can (which is sometimes done in other countries), and that the beans or other foods are packed in water and are sodium free. When you're ready to use the canned food, drain the contents to remove excess salt.

WHOLE GRAINS

Grains and cereals are rich sources of vitamins, minerals, carbohydrates, fats, oils, and protein in their whole grain form. Quinoa and amaranth aren't actually grains, but pseudocereals, broadleaf plants that are prepared similarly to grains. All of the grains listed on the next page are gluten-free, with the exception of barley, which is used in one recipe in this book. Furthermore, oats are technically gluten-free, but they are typically packaged with other grains that contain gluten, so cross-contamination is practically unavoidable. Look for oats that are labeled gluten-free. Most grains last up to three months when stored in an airtight glass container in a dark, cool pantry.

- Amaranth
- Barley
- Brown rice
- Black rice
- Corn grits
- Quinoa
- Millet
- Oats, gluten-free
- Steel-cut oats
- Yam noodles

FLOUR MIXES AND BAKING MATERIALS

In keeping with the gluten-free recipes, there is no wheat flour used in this cookbook's recipes. Below are recommended gluten-free alternatives. Feel free to swap or alternate any wheat-free flour for any others in these recipes.

- Arrowroot flour
- Brown rice flour
- Buckwheat flour
- Chickpea flour
- Cornmeal
- Kudzu flour
- Potato flour
- Quinoa flour
- Tapioca flour
- White rice flour

NON-DAIRY PRODUCTS

There are plenty of non-dairy milk and yogurt options available in stores, and there is also a recipe for making your own on page 62! Here are some healthy choices.

- Almond milk
- Coconut milk
- Hemp milk
- Soy milk
- Live-culture coconut yogurt
- Live-culture soy yogurt

OILS

There is much to say on the subject of oils. First of all, oils do not store well for long periods of time. Do your best and try to get your oils as fresh as possible, with at least a one-year expiration date—and then try to use the entire bottle within two months and replace.

Secondly, make sure you are choosing fats that will do the most good for your health and longevity. Stay clear of saturated animal fats, such as butter and lard, which cause inflammation and elevate cholesterol and triglyceride levels. The key to preventing heart disease and inflammation is to choose polyunsaturated fats with omega-3 fatty acids, such as extra-virgin olive oil. These fats help your body maintain a healthy balance of cholesterol. The oils that I recommend are listed on the opposite page, and like everything else, they should be used in moderation.

Also, you need to consider each oil's smoke point, the temperature at which oil begins to break down—which creates a chemical change in the oil that is harmful to eat. It is very important to not heat oil past its smoke point. You can tell you have reached the smoke point when you begin to see gaseous vapors coming from the heated oil.

- High smoke point oils include avocado oil, rice bran oil, and grapeseed oil. Use these oils if you are planning on roasting, sautéing, baking, or otherwise heating your oil hotter than 275°F.
- Medium smoke point oils include olive oil, walnut oil, and sesame oil. These oils will work nicely for making flavorful sauces or for lightly simmering food, but their smoke point is usually not high enough for sautéing, depending on how highly refined the oil is. The more refined the oil, the higher the smoke point—but since unrefined oil has more nutrients, I recommend choosing unrefined over refined oil and cooking with it at lower temperatures.
- Fish oil, flaxseed oil, and hemp oil are very beneficial for your heart and overall health but are not intended for cooking. Simply drizzle these oils over your prepared food.

SAUCES, STOCKS, AND SPREADS

In general, I think it is best to make sauces, stocks, and spreads from scratch, especially since prepackaged versions of these foods can be high in sodium and other unhealthy additives. Also, as previously mentioned, canned food can be high in sodium and the cans may be lined with BPA, so if you're buying packaged food, it's best to purchase food sold in glass jars. Below are several sauces, stocks, and spreads that show up in longevity recipes.

- Tomato sauce, tomato puree, and tomato paste
- Low-sodium chicken stock
- Marinated artichoke hearts
- Sesame tahini
- Marmalade preserves
- Peanut butter

VINEGARS, CONDIMENTS, AND FLAVORINGS

Vinegar is a very healthy food in its own right, and it also adds a unique, delicious flavor to other foods. Vinegar and these other condiments will help bring your food alive with flavor. The alcohol is for cooking—a small amount of wine in a tasty soup can add just the right amount of zest!

- Rice vinegar
- Red wine vinegar
- Apple cider vinegar
- Light soy sauce (low-sodium, gluten-free, and MSG-free)
- Dark soy sauce (low-sodium, gluten-free, and MSG-free)
- Chili bean sauce
- Miso paste (low-sodium and MSG-free)
- Tamari
- Chicken bouillon
- Pickled organic cucumber (low-sodium)
- Pickled ginger
- Port
- Sake
- Sherry
- White wine

SWEETENERS

Below are the natural sweeteners that I recommend for baking and other sweet recipes. Even though these sweeteners are far healthier than refined sugar, they should still be used in moderation.

- Stevia is the best sweetener in my opinion, because it is a plant-based sweetener with no calories and will not upset blood glucose levels.
- Honey, especially local wildflower honey
- Maple syrup
- Brown rice syrup
- Malt sugar
- Molasses
- Diced dried fruits or dates—sprinkle these into your baked goods and they will add natural sweetness without upsetting sugar balance in your body.
- Cinnamon is a fantastic sweetener in tea and baked dishes. Cinnamon contributes to a healthy balance of blood sugar, helping to balance and treat diabetes.

DRIED FRUITS

Below are the dried fruits that I often include in trail mixes, warm cereal, or in baking in place of sugar. When purchasing dried fruit, look for unsweetened (or no sugar added) dried fruit.

- Apricots, dried
- Blueberries, dried
- California dried plums (prunes)
- Cranberries, dried
- Figs, dried
- Goji berries
- Papaya, dried, sulfite-free if possible
- Pineapple, dried, sulfite-free if possible

Dried Foods

Drying foods does not destroy the foods' nutrients, although in fruits, certain vitamins can be easily lost. Vitamin C, for instance, is fragile, so it may be destroyed in the dehydration process. That is one reason why fruits are generally better fresh. Otherwise, dried foods are nearly as beneficial as the fresh versions, which is helpful if you would like to use an unusual mushroom or seaweed in a new recipe. To reconstitute dried foods, you simply soak them in water until they plump up to their original size and then cook with them as you usually would. Store dried foods in airtight glass containers. Keep in mind that dried foods will not last forever and the nutrient levels in the foods will degrade over time. It's important to note that frozen foods retain their nutrients better than dried foods.

DRIED SPECIALTY ITEMS

Fresh seaweed and out-of-season mushrooms are most easily found in ethnic or specialty food stores. Dried versions of these foods can also be found in larger chain stores. If fresh shiitake mushrooms happen to be available, buy those over the dried variety. Here are dried specialty items that frequently come up in this cookbook's longevity recipes.

- Hijiki seaweed
- Kombu seaweed
- Nori seaweed
- Wakame seaweed

- Porcini mushrooms
- Shiitake mushrooms
- Wood ear mushrooms

HERBS AND SPICES

With their incredible flavors and amazing healing properties, herbs and spices bring out the best in longevity cooking! A variety of herbs and spices will also help you put down the salt shaker, which is welcoming news for your heart. Store dried herbs and spices in airtight glass jars in a dark place. The volatile oils in herbs and spices, which are responsible for their healing abilities, will eventually evaporate, taking all the beneficial properties with them. When bottled spices aren't giving off much of a fragrance, it's time to toss them—typically six to twelve months. I personally use plenty of herbs and spices, so my supplies typically run out before their expiration dates, and I hope it is the same for you! If you happen to have a spice grinder or mortar and pestle, consider buying these herbs whole, such as coriander or cardamom pods, and grind them yourself just before eating, to preserve the volatile oils. When a recipe calls for fresh herbs, it is best to use a freshly picked variety rather than dried.

Essential Spices

These are the essential herbs and spices for longevity cooking that come up most frequently in these recipes.

- Black pepper
- Cardamom, ground
- Cayenne pepper
- Cinnamon, ground
- Cinnamon sticks
- Cloves, ground
- Cloves, whole
- Ginger, ground
- Paprika
- Red chili flakes
- Sea salt
- Turmeric, ground

Grow Your Own
Healthy, growing herbs are a wonderful, aromatic addition to your kitchen. Why not fill your kitchen with potted herbs for easy access while you cook? Some of the easier-to-grow herbs for a sunny window include basil, rosemary, sage, dill, mint, and parsley.

Other Delightful Spices

- Anise
- Bay leaves
- Coriander, ground
- Cumin, ground
- Curry powder
- Fennel, ground
- Garlic powder
- Parsley
- Rosemary
- Saffron threads
- Sage
- Star anise
- Thyme
- White pepper
- Masala spice (ground cumin, cinnamon, clove, bay leaf, peppercorn, coriander, cardamom)

EXOTIC HERBS AND SUPPLEMENTS

Some of the longevity recipes in this book call for powerful, exotic herbs that may be challenging to find. Some of these herbs may be purchased online; just make sure you are buying from a reputable purveyor. Also, some health-food stores and Asian markets may carry these specialty items. You will find most of these herbs already dried or ground. Where helpful, I have included the Asian names, as well as English names. These herbs truly are the heart of many longevity recipes—and the unparalleled healing benefits should not be missed!

- Angelica root (Dang gui)
- Atractylodis (Bai zhu)
- Five Elements Greens Powder, available on Ask Dr. Mao site
- Fox nut
- Ginseng (Ren sheng)
- Hemp powder
- High Performance Powder, available on Ask Dr. Mao site
- Kelp powder
- Licorice (Gan cao)
- Lily blossom
- Lily bulb
- Ligustici (Chuang xiong)
- Lotus root
- Lotus seed
- Poria (Fu ling)
- Red jujube date
- Rehmannia (Shou di)
- White peony (Shao yao)
- Wild yam root

Using traditional Chinese medicine as our guide, my staff and I have created pre-mixed spice blends to support a variety of conditions, including improving heart health, boosting immunity, countering inflammation, and increasing metabolism. You can mix these spice blends yourself, but if you don't happen to have a wide variety of spices and herbs in your cupboards or the time to grind and mix them, you will be happy to know that you can easily purchase them through the Ask Dr. Mao site. See page 47 for more spice blend recipes.

FREEZING FOOD: PRESERVE THE NUTRIENTS AND SAVE FOR LATER

Water is the main element of fresh, whole food, usually making up between 50 to 90 percent of the natural food's weight. Freezing is an excellent way to main-tain these water levels and temporarily stop the growth of microorganisms and bacteria. In general, freezing food doesn't lessen nutritional value if you freeze the food when it is at peak quality. For example, if berries are flash frozen as soon as they're picked, there's very little loss of nutritional value. In fact, nutrients are better retained in frozen fruits and vegetables than in those "fresh" varieties that are transported long distances to their destination. Produce begins to lose valuable vitamins and minerals soon after being picked, especially at room temperature and warmer. Freezing fresh produce for a few hours after harvesting can help prevent this nutritional loss.

If you have a large portion of produce on your hands from your summer garden or local farmer's market, you should consider freezing your fruits and vegetables for later use. Using a vacuum sealer or wrapping your foods in several layers of waxed paper or butcher paper can help avoid freezer burn. Storebought flash-frozen fruit and vegetables are also great additions to stir-fry recipes or other main dishes.

Label your frozen items with the date they were frozen and when to use them by, usually between three and six months. Make sure the foods you freeze—whether vegetables, fruit, nuts, meats—are fresh and unspoiled before you freeze them. You'll want to freeze everything in meal-sized portions, as it can be difficult to separate portions once frozen.

Smart Shopping Tips for Longevity

Now that you know what foods to buy, it's time to get busy at the supermarket, health-food store, and farmer's market. Here are some tips to easily navigate your local grocery store for health and longevity.

- **Make a Game Plan.** Create a menu plan for the entire week and write a detailed shopping list of what you'll need so you won't impulsively toss an unhealthy product into your cart.
- **Never Shop on an Empty Stomach.** If you do, you may leave the store with more items (some not so healthy) than you originally planned on!
- **Shop the Edge of Glory.** Superfoods meant for health and longevity mainly live along the perimeter of the grocery store. These foods include fruit, vegetables, organic meats and eggs that are antibiotic- and hormone-free, fish, tofu, and often your milk alternatives, like soy milk. Items you find in the inner aisles of the market tend to be boxed, canned, or processed foods. A few exceptions might include bags of dried beans, legumes, nuts, and seeds.

Essential Utensils and Cookware for Longevity

The longevity recipes in this cookbook will help you stay healthy and prevent disease, but not if you use the wrong supplies in your food preparation and cooking techniques. Some containers and utensils may leach toxic substances and change properties of your food—at the very least, downgrading the nutrition, and more seriously, actually causing you harm. As in everything else, I recommend adopting an attitude of moderation. Control what you can within your kitchen and be relaxed while eating at a friend's house or in restaurants. Stay informed and do your research—make sure your kitchen contains only the safest, most trusted utensils and cookware. Read on for some of my personal thoughts in regard to cookware and kitchen utensils.

COOKWARE: BEST OPTIONS

Porcelain-Lined Enamel Cookware

As far as I am concerned, porcelain-lined enamel cookware is the ideal cooking container. Enameled cookware is made of heavy metal, usually cast iron, which is then coated with enamel. This type of cookware is nonstick and very durable. It should last more than a lifetime if properly cared for—so think of these pots as an investment in your family's health, which can be passed down to your children. To care for your enamel cookware, allow it to completely cool before hand washing with warm soapy water and a sponge. Do not use abrasive cleaning tools or harsh chemicals because they may damage the enamel. Also, avoid using metal utensils with this cookware, which can also chip and damage the enamel.

Glassware and CorningWare

Glassware is wonderful for cooking, but it can be hard to find a suitably sturdy glass pot. First introduced in 1958 and now making a resurgence in American households, CorningWare was originally a brand name for a pyroceramic glass cookware that was created to resist thermal shock. CorningWare is notable for the fact that it can be used directly on the stovetop as well as in the oven.

Cast Iron

Overall, cast iron is a very sturdy and dependable type of cookware. Its only downside is that it can leach iron into your food, which for some people is not a problem if they suffer from an iron deficiency, but in general, too much iron is not healthy for your body. Cast iron skillets are excellent for searing in flavor and also for baking. Cast iron cookware is easily cleaned with a damp paper towel and very little soap. A well-seasoned cast iron pan can last for decades.

Terra-Cotta Clay Pot

A clay cooker is a vessel that promotes the slow evaporation of steam when food is saturated with water and heated in the oven, creating a moist, enclosed environment that results in intense flavor and tender, healthy food. Traditional clay cooking pots come from all over the world, from the *tagine* in Morocco, the *cazuela* in Spain, sand pots from China, and tandoor pots from India. Look for a lead-free terra-cotta clay pot. Follow the manufacturer's instructions regarding the correct cooking and cleaning methods for each pot.

Stainless Steel

While stainless steel is generally safe to cook with, stainless steel cookware may start leaching nickel, zinc, copper, and other types of metals into your food if scrubbed too vigorously with an abrasive sponge or powder. If you own stainless steel cookware, watch your cooking temperatures to make sure you don't overheat the pans, since they are less sturdy than some of the other cookware previously described. When cleaning your stainless steel pots and pans, soak them overnight with lemon juice and vinegar, and avoid using harsh detergents or chemicals.

COOKWARE: WORST OPTIONS

Nonstick Pans

Although nonstick pans are handy in the kitchen, they contain unnatural chemical, and plastic components that have been linked to immune disorders and possible cancer conditions. Improved cooking techniques with other, safer cookware can easily mirror the benefits of nonstick pans, such as simply making sure your pans are well-oiled and well-seasoned.

Aluminum and Copper Cookware

Aluminum and copper interact with heat, and traces of these harmful metals can potentially leak into your food. Gradually these metals will accumulate in your body, sometimes reaching the point of toxicity. Toxic levels of aluminum have been linked to memory loss, headaches, indigestion, and brain disorders, including Alzheimer's disease. High levels of copper can debilitate the immune system and enable cancer cells to proliferate. It's important to note however, that if used sparingly, copper and aluminum shouldn't be a health risk for most people.

Baking Sheets

When baking, I recommend forgoing nonstick baking sheets and aluminum foil for oven-safe CorningWare or enamel cookware, which are both essentially nonstick alternatives.

COOKING UTENSILS

Plastic spatulas may seep polychlorinated biphenyls (PCBs), phthalates, or other toxic chemicals into your food. Such leaching occurs even more when utensils are washed and rewashed in high-temperature dishwashers. If you can, avoid using plastic utensils and storage containers.

Wood and bamboo are absolutely the best options for spatulas, spoons, and other utensils. Wood and bamboo will not transfer any potentially harmful chemicals into your food and they are gentle on enamel cookware and other cookware. Stainless steel utensils are your next best option. Steel is very easy to clean and its unique surface has no pores or cracks to harbor dirt, grime, or bacteria, though, as previously mentioned, stainless steel can cause some issues related to leaching when scrubbed too vigorously.

DISH DOS

Always use lead-free, high-quality, ceramic dishware and drink out of glassware, not plastic cups. A fun money-saving tip is to save and rinse out glass jars that contain jam, olives, or other items after use for your family's primary drinking glasses.

STORAGE SOLUTIONS

Replace all plastic storage containers with glass containers. The best choices are those that are made completely of glass, including glass lids. Mason jars and glass containers with metal caps or plastic lids (BPA- and PVC-free) are acceptable, as long as the food is not in long-term contact with the lids. Instead of plastic wrap or bags, use butcher paper wrap, parchment paper, or unbleached waxed paper bags.

Not convinced this action is worth the effort? Simply flip over your plastic food storage containers and look at the number printed on the bottom. If the recycling number is #3, #6, or #7, steer clear! These items likely contain bisphenol A (BPA), an endocrine disrupter that disturbs hormonal balance; polystyrene (PS), a suspected carcinogen, thought to be toxic for gastrointestinal, kidney, and respiratory systems; or phthalates (used to make PVC plastics) which mimic estrogen and can interfere with hormone levels. These plastics can also seep into food, particularly when warmed up in the microwave or washed at high heat in the dishwasher.

MICROWAVES: DESTROY NUTRIENTS

Although microwaves certainly are convenient for our busy schedules, you might want to reconsider using the one in your kitchen. Microwave ovens work by using a form of radiation—waves of electrical and magnetic energy—to make molecules in the food rotate and move, producing heat. (It uses a non-ionizing electromagnetic radiation and not particle radiation, like ultraviolet or x-rays.) Not only has microwave use been linked to causing infertility in men, one study by the Spanish scientific research council known as CEBAS-CSIC, which was published in the *Journal of the Science of Food and Agriculture,* found that microwave cooking destroys some important nutrients in vegetables. Microwaved broccoli lost over 75 percent of three cancer-protecting antioxidants compared to steamed broccoli, which lost just over 10 percent of these compounds.

If you must cook food in your microwave, use the low setting to heat food, and use only glassware, CorningWare, ceramic, or lead-free terra-cotta bowls. A safer option for heating up your food is to use a small toaster oven or steam oven. This method may take more time, but it is much healthier for your food and for you.

HELPFUL KITCHEN TOOLS

There are a few other key tools that will enhance your cooking experience and that will come in handy when you prepare recipes from this book.

Wok

A wok makes stir-frying a breeze and is a fun, useful addition to any kitchen.

Crockpot or Slow Cooker

Crockpots and slow cookers can save you a great deal of time that would otherwise be spent over the stove, particularly with beans, soups, cereals, and anything else that requires more than two hours of cooking. Even better, slow cooking helps you get the biggest nutritious bang from your healthy foods by helping you digest them better. When you are bloated, it is often because your digestive system is having trouble breaking down the food you just ate, be it beans, legumes, or other food. Slow cooking does some of the heavy lifting for your digestive system by helping to break down the outer cellulose layer of beans and legumes, which also helps release the food's nutrients for your body to more easily absorb.

Blender and Juicer

A blender is indispensable for smoothies. I personally use a bullet blender, which has a serving size meant for one person. Fresh juices do not play a major role in this cookbook, but they are incredibly useful tools nonetheless. Juices are particularly potent and powerful when they include plenty of fresh vegetables and seaweed, so you may want to invest in a juicer as well. Juicers help process the nutrients from the juice so it's easier for the body to absorb—but a blender will work similarly.

Spice grinder

A spice grinder—or a coffee grinder that is used just for grinding spices—will save you loads of time if you love to cook with plenty of dried spices in their whole form, such as cardamom pods and peppercorns. Make sure you grind spices right before adding them to your dish, in order to release the aromas and preserve the healthy volatile oils.

Proper Prep and Safe Cleaning

Now that you have the correct utensils for cooking healthy meals, make sure to also use safe and healthy preparation and cleaning methods in the kitchen.

USE TWO CUTTING BOARDS

When you chop and dice food, use two cutting boards, ideally made of wood. Reserve one for produce only, and the other for animal products. Cutting vegetables on the same board as raw chicken or other meats will increase the chance of cross-contamination of bacteria, such as salmonella. After each use, clean the board by hand with warm water and dish soap. Select phosphorus-free natural cleaning dish soap; it will not leave chemical residue on your board. Cleaning will not fully sterilize the board per se, but it will keep bacteria, viruses, and parasites from sticking to the board. The point of using dish soap is to unstick everything, including bacteria from the cutting surface. Periodically, you may pour hydrogen peroxide on the surface, let it sit for one minute, and wash off.

PRODUCE CLEANING POINTERS

You may not be able to tell by looking at your fruits and vegetables, but they are often covered with pesticides, wax, possibly bacteria, and whatever else they came in contact with when transported, sorted, and placed in the market bins. Make sure you carefully wash all produce before eating! Organic produce will be less likely to have unhealthy coatings, but it is still an excellent rule of thumb to wash all fruits and vegetables before eating. If you like, you can use the natural produce wash found in health-food stores. Salt also works as a natural sterilizer. When I come home with a big bounty of fresh produce, I use a colander nestled inside a larger bowl, add water and salt, then I douse my produce in the water and rinse it off a few times. To clean leafy greens, fill up the sink with cold water and let them soak to loosen the dirt that clings to the leaves. Drain the sink and repeat the same steps until the water runs clear. Remove the greens and spin or pat them dry before storing them in the refrigerator. For root vegetables, citrus fruits, and harder-skinned produce, you can use a gentle scrubbing brush to clean.

KEEP YOUR KITCHEN SPARKLING NATURALLY

Toss out the toxic cleaning products and go back to basics. These days, there is an abundance of natural cleaning products on the market, which are safe and will bring cleanliness to your kitchen without putting toxins in the environment or your home. It's also very easy to make your own home cleaning products! Diluted vinegar is an effective, natural kitchen cleanser. Just mix 1 cup of distilled white vinegar with 1 cup of water and use as you would any cleaning product. Vinegar also inhibits the growth of bacteria and mildew, which is a plus for your countertops or other often-used surfaces. Baking soda can be sprinkled on your stovetop, left for a few minutes and then scoured with a scrubber. For the stubborn spots that refuse to go away, try this: mix dishwashing liquid, borax, and warm water, spray and let sit for twenty minutes, and then scour the surface.

EATING AND COOKING FOR LONGEVITY

"To avoid sickness, eat less; to prolong life, worry less."

—CHU HUI WENG

In the previous section, you learned *what* centenarians eat. In this section, I want to share with you *how* centenarians eat and how they approach food preparation. You will learn the top ten centenarian rules for eating, which I learned when I interviewed and studied the habits of centenarians and which I've used in my own practice of traditional Chinese medicine.

We need to relearn these golden rules of centenarian eating because we typically prioritize quick, cheap, and easy over fulfilling, wholesome, and nutritious. We also have the tendency to eat at unhealthy times, such as consuming a plate of greasy food right before bed—or we rush through meals, as if eating is an inconvenience keeping us from a more important agenda. But what is more important than eating? You can't live without food! And more importantly, you can't live very well without nutritious, wholesome foods! In many parts of the world, life revolves around food, from the creative and giving aspect of preparing meals to the communal sharing of the food. Those who value food—preparing, cooking, and sharing it—benefit from a better quality of life, a better quality of nutrition, and a longer, more fulfilled life. With this book, I seek to change the tides of unhealthy eating in the U.S. I sincerely wish to remake food into the communal, nutritious life force it once was in our country.

It's time to change our eating and cooking habits for the better, and this process does not have to be agonizingly difficult. With a few adjustments and lifestyle improvements, you will not only be on the road to longevity, but you will also find more enjoyment and zest in your life than you ever did before embarking on this exciting journey!

Top Ten Longevity Habits
for Good Digestion and Good Health

Of what benefit is it to eat healthy, antioxidant-rich foods if your body is not able to digest them properly? Proper digestion is essential to living a long and healthy life. Your body's digestive tract is made up of numerous organs that work together to break down, absorb, and process all of the nutrients in the food you consume. When digestive function is disrupted, bloating, gas, weight gain, fatigue, constipation or diarrhea, and abdominal pain ensue. Without healthy digestion, you can become malnourished and toxins can build up in your body, leading to degenerative diseases and more rapid aging.

Indigestion is caused by and worsened due to overeating—particularly rich, fatty, excessively sugary and salty foods, alcohol, coffee, and other acidic foods. Eating balanced portions of healthy foods along with the right food preparation are the keys to overcoming debilitating digestive issues. These ten time-tested longevity golden rules will keep your digestion and overall health on the right track.

CENTENARIAN HABIT #1: EAT LESS TO LIVE LONGER

For generations, many centenarians have come from very modest means, and as a consequence, they often ate smaller meals. This tradition continues today as centenarians typically eat smaller portions than other adults. They eat only until their stomachs are three-quarters full, a far cry from the super-sized portions of most meals today. When you overeat, you stress your digestive and other organ systems, consuming precious energy by overworking your system, and producing more waste products and toxins. Eating less improves your overall digestion by boosting metabolism and allowing you to absorb more nutrients from your food. Many studies show that calorie restriction—or eating less food—increases lifespan in animals. On the other hand, excess animal protein has been found to increase the risk of cancer and kidney disease, and excess fat leads to obesity and higher risk of heart disease and stroke.

Try to control the amount of food you eat at each meal by stopping when your stomach is three-quarters full. Many of the dishes in this book are smaller portions, and the recipes are meant to help train you so you will be satisfied and happy when you are just three-quarters full. Enjoy your food, but a little at a time!

CENTENARIAN HABIT #2: EAT FIVE SMALLER MEALS A DAY

Most of us are accustomed to eating three large meals a day, but this is a cultural habit. It is much healthier to eat smaller meals more frequently over the course of the day. I personally recommend eating five small meals a day. Eating in this way delivers a steady stream of nutrients, blood sugar, and energy to your body throughout the day and is much less taxing on the digestive and metabolic systems than eating large, heavy meals. Also, when you eat more small meals throughout the day, you will most likely avoid the pitfalls of overindulging at your next meal—helping you consume fewer total calories for the day.

CENTENARIAN HABIT #3: EAT YOUR MEALS ON TIME

It is true that "you are what you eat," but it is also true that "you are *when* you eat." The human body follows a circadian rhythm, and as a result, the same foods eaten at breakfast and lunch are processed differently than when eaten at dinnertime. Studies have shown that when you consume your daily protein and fat earlier in the day, you tend to lose weight and have more energy. On the other hand, eating the same protein and fat late in the evening tends to increase risks of weight gain, high blood pressure, and heart disease. This truth is why I often say "eat like a king by day, like a pauper by night." Most importantly, never eat right before bedtime unless you want your stomach to be working all night long!

Your body functions best when fed at regular intervals. As a general rule, I suggest eating your meals during these times.

- **Breakfast** should be eaten between 6:00 and 9:00 a.m.
- A **mid-morning snack** can come between 10:30 and 11:00 a.m.
- **Lunch** should be between 12:00 and 1:30 p.m.
- A **mid-afternoon snack** can come between 3:00 and 4:00 p.m.
- **Dinner** should be eaten between 6:00 and 7:30 p.m.

CENTENARIAN HABIT #4: EAT SLOWLY AND ENJOY YOUR FOOD

Most of us eat too quickly, putting an unnecessary burden on our digestive system. As I often tell my patients, your stomach does not have teeth! The digestive process, particularly the digestion of starches, begins in the mouth where enzymes are produced to help break down and absorb nutrients. Help your digestive system do its job well by chewing each bite twenty times and savoring the flavor. Foods that are difficult to thoroughly masticate, such as flaxseeds and sesame seeds, should be ground before eating.

Eating too quickly can easily lead to eating too much. It takes roughly twenty minutes for your brain to signal your stomach that it's full, yet by that time, you may have already eaten enough dinner for two people if you haven't taken your time to enjoy your food! If you have developed a habit of briskly wolfing down your food, slow down with these tricks:

- Put your fork or spoon down between each bite to give you more time to chew.
- Drink a glass of water before each meal—this practice will help you feel more full, so that you will be less inclined to ravenously attack your plate.
- Eating should be about sharing special moments with friends and loved ones. Enjoy meals as a family and spend more time indulging in conversation and less on food.

CENTENARIAN HABIT #5: TAKE YOUR MEALS SITTING DOWN

Centenarians are often very hard workers, but they also know the importance of sitting down and enjoying a meal when it is time to eat. Do not eat at your computer. Do not eat while you are running to your next appointment. Do not eat in your car. Focus on the flavor and texture of the food, sit down at the table, and interact with others during your meal. This way you will not overeat, you will enjoy your meal more heartily, and your food will be more easily digested.

CENTENARIAN HABIT #6: EAT FOR YOUR BODY, NOT YOUR TASTE BUDS

They may make your tongue happy, but high-calorie processed snacks will never fully satisfy your body's need for critical nutrients. You will feel healthier and more energetic if you eat for nutrition instead of immediate pleasure. You have the power to choose what you put into your mouth. Before eating, ask yourself if your food choices will positively contribute to your health and well-being or if they will cause future problems and discomfort. A lot of people "live to eat" instead of "eating to live"—they eat lavishly and decadently, falsely fulfilling their bellies in place of their hearts. Eat to *thrive*, like centenarians who have lived well past 100 and rarely touch salty, sugary snacks!

CENTENARIAN HABIT #7: EAT FOR THE RIGHT REASONS

Centenarians mainly eat only when they are hungry. That statement may sound obvious, but think of how many empty calories we consume in any given day simply because we walk by a tasty-looking treat, or a co-worker offers us a sugary snack. We sometimes eat out of habit at a certain time of day without realizing that we are not even hungry. Before eating anything, ask yourself: would you eat an apple, a banana, or a vegetable instead? If the answer is no, then you're not actually hungry. If the answer is yes, listen to your body and eat healthy foods to thrive!

CENTENARIAN HABIT #8: BRING AWARENESS TO MEALTIME

In many traditional centenarian cultures, it is customary to say a prayer over the food before eating. Such a meditation practice does not have to be a prayer—simply take a pause before you eat to recognize that the food is providing your body with necessary nutrients and energy. Even this brief moment will set the tone for a mindful, peaceful meal, which will help you stay more relaxed and help your body digest your food more easily. Refrain from eating if you are nervous or upset. Eating in a relaxed frame of mind is essential to proper digestion and assimilation of nutrients. Even better, regularly eating lovingly prepared meals with friends and family members will help all those at the table feel more at ease and fulfilled in life.

Be Prepared to Eat on the Go

You may not always have time to cook all of your own meals, but you can take steps so that you don't make poor, unhealthy choices when you're out and about.

- Instead of chips or sugary snacks, get your crunch from fresh vegetables. Hummus is a complementary snack that travels well and is packed with protein, so it's perfect to eat between meals with fresh vegetables.
- Satisfy your sweet tooth with fresh fruit, instead of a high-calorie muffin or a sugary treat. Apples, oranges, peaches, cherries, and bananas are delicious choices that can be sliced and brought along to work or weekend activities.
- Stave off hunger between meals and keep your energy high with protein-packed trail mix. Combine nuts, seeds, and dried fruits in waxed paper bags to bring on the go.
- Avoid fatty fast food with a satisfying lunch or snack at the ready. Brown rice with pine nuts and steamed vegetables is a small, light meal that is easy to pack in a lidded mason jar.

CENTENARIAN HABIT #9: EAT FOOD AT THE PROPER TEMPERATURE TO SUPPORT YOUR DIGESTIVE FIRE

In many healing traditions, such as traditional Chinese medicine and India's Ayurvedic medicine, it is taught that cold, icy foods and beverages put out the digestive fire. Your body's temperature is around 98.6 degrees, and ice cream or cold iced beverages are often around 30 degrees. Imagine if you ran outside in a near-freezing temperature with no clothes on. How do you think your body would react? Likewise, the shock your digestive tract experiences from the sudden drop in temperature from cold foods may cause gastric juice imbalance, decreased blood flow in your stomach, and painful spasms in the bowels, among many other uncomfortable side effects. For this reason, avoid icy foods and try to eat foods at room temperatures or close to your body's own temperature.

Even chilled and raw salads are recommended only in moderation, as they are also thought to be more difficult to digest than room-temperature food. Traditional Chinese medicine practitioners believe that cooking your food adds warming energy, which is then in turn supportive to your digestion. As previously described, cooking food thoroughly also helps break its nutrients down so it's easier for your body to digest them without your stomach having to do the heavy labor.

Get Smart About Eating Out

Ideally, you would always be able to cook at home, where you can control exactly what goes into your meals. Of course, it is not always possible to eat at home every-day, and furthermore, going out to eat with friends and family members can be a fun occasion. Here are some helpful tips for these occasions:

- Choose restaurants that are nutrition-oriented. Avoid fast-food restaurants or diners serving only fried, fatty foods. On the menu, the vegetarian fare is usually the healthiest option, as long as it is fresh and not fried.
- Plated portions in restaurants are almost always more than our bodies need. Your body can only make use of a certain amount of nutrients at a given time. Try choosing an appetizer, a soup, or a salad for lunch instead of an entrée, which is almost always too much food for one person. One or two of these smaller dishes can fill you up and give you some variety, without leaving you overstuffed and lethargic.
- If you do order an entrée, ask for a box when it arrives and box up half of the portion before you start eating. That way, you won't be tempted to finish the whole plate.
- Eating with a close friend or family member? Offer to split the entrée order.

CENTENARIAN HABIT #10: EVERYTHING IN MODERATION

Keep in mind that you can eat for longevity without completely sacrificing your favorite treats. The occasional glass of wine, slice of birthday cake, or rich appetizer isn't going to ruin your health, as long as you are moderate in your approach and mindful of portion size. Most of the time, just a small bite is enough to satisfy your taste buds. Keep these portion guidelines in mind: 4 to 5 ounces of meat is the size of a deck of cards; ½ cup of rice is the size of a light bulb; 1 ounce of cheese equals the size of 3 stacked dice. Enjoy a small sample of the foods you love and don't go back for seconds. Everything in moderation!

Eat for Your Body's Unique Needs

By listening to your body and understanding your own needs, you can choose the appropriate foods to bring about a balanced state of health. All foods have inherent healing qualities. Based on these qualities, foods are broadly categorized into hot and warming, cold and cooling, and neutral (which is neither hot nor cold). In general, animal products like poultry, meat, eggs, and dairy are warming, while vegetables, fruits, and liquids are cooling. Whole grains, beans, legumes, deep-sea fish, and most nuts and seeds are neutral. There are exceptions to this rule, such as cherries, which are considered warming, even though they are a fruit. Pork is cooling, even though it is an animal product.

Use these principles to help you eat for the season and to help you find balance in your diet. The dog days of summer are an appropriate time to eat salads and vegetables with cooling properties. When we're in the midst of cold winter weather, you should support your body with warm teas and hearty soups. Also, use these principles to eat for your particular body's needs. To keep it simple, let's just talk about the two main constitutional types.

HOT TYPE—OVER-DRIVE

If you overheat easily, frequently have a dry mouth and red face, easily lose your temper, are regularly thirsty, urinate infrequently, and are often constipated, you are a hot type. You would counteract your hot type imbalance by eating a cooling diet with raw vegetables and salads, and by choosing cooling foods like cucumber, watermelon, and peppermint. You may also need to eat less protein such as red meat and poultry.

COLD TYPE—UNDER-DRIVE

If you are a person who tends to be often chilly, is often tired, runs to the restroom frequently, has a hard time losing weight, tends toward depression, has a pale complexion and perhaps foul-smelling stools, then you are a cold type. Warming foods such as ginger, roasted chestnut, and fenugreek may be helpful for you, and you are better off avoiding raw foods like salad. Soups, hot tea, and eating more animal products will help balance your cold nature. While vegetables and fruits are in the cold foods category, they are fine for a cold type to eat if they are cooked, as the cooking process neutralizes the cold properties.

So, how do you figure out what your personal needs are and what your balanced diet should be? First, you must discover whether your body is in over-drive or under-drive—hot or cold, respectively. Which of the above descriptions most fits you? If you don't match either description, but in fact, have a steady temperament, have a normal-colored complexion, and have regular bowel movements, you may already be in balance. If this subject is of interest to you, I recommend finding a traditional Chinese medical practitioner to get more in-depth advice about your own body and specific diet needs.

On your own, a helpful way to know what works for your individual needs is to pay close attention to the reactions you have to food. Try keeping a food journal for a few days to record how food affects you. Maybe you notice that you feel bloated not long after eating a raw salad or lethargic after eating a big meal. Make note of these things, put them to the test a few times (unless they cause immediate illness, of course), and make adjustments according to your dietary needs and reactions. The overall take-home message is that this process is about keeping balance in your body—eating what your body needs is the key to longevity!

Food Preparation Methods to Support Longevity

When making your food for longevity, not all preparation methods are of equal benefit! Many of the food preparation methods Americans often use to add intense flavor, such frying and grilling, may seem tasty to your tongue, but are definitely not beneficial to your stomach or overall health. The list that follows covers most food preparation methods, from best to worst.

• **Steaming** is the best cooking method because it preserves the integrity of the food's nutrients better than any other method. With less heat, you won't risk denaturing the proteins or fats in your food.

• **Stir-frying** or stewing in water over low heat is another cooking method that loses minimal amounts of nutritional value. For several dishes in this book, I recommend putting a little water in your cooking pan, heating the pan to a sizzle, then tossing in produce to steam-cook vegetables for a few minutes. Once the vegetables are cooked, you can turn off the heat and then add a bit of oil. This method preserves the most nutrients in your food and keeps the oil in its healthiest state.

• **Stir-frying** with oil is acceptable as long as you stir-fry food quickly and use the oils with the highest smoke points, which can withstand higher temperatures up to 400°F before being destroyed and becoming carcinogenic. Grapeseed, rice bran, and avocado oils are the oils that I use most often for stir-frying.

• **Baking and roasting at low temperatures** will also preserve nutrients to some extent. Baking and roasting at higher temperatures is fine from a safety standpoint as long as you don't burn any food and you use high smoke point oils. Remember, anything cooked until it is black can be carcinogenic, so keep a close eye on whatever you are cooking. Also, in general, the higher the cooking temperature, the more nutrients may be destroyed in the cooking process.

• **Grilling** may be a fun outdoor activity, but it is not the best cooking method. Again, anytime food is blackened or burnt, it can be very difficult on your digestive system and even potentially carcinogenic. Eating grilled food once in a while is not harmful to your health, but you should avoid eating anything black and burnt.

• **Deep-frying in fat** is the worst method for preparing food. In addition to adding very high levels of fat to your food and therefore canceling out health benefits, most individuals don't use the appropriate oil for frying at such a high temperature, which denatures the structure of the oil, which can potentially be carcinogenic. As previously noted, cooking with high heat destroys the nutrients in your food. If you must deep-fry in fat, use the best quality oil with the highest heating point.

• **Microwaving food** is also a poor cooking method since it strips nutrients from food. See additional details regarding microwave cooking on page 33.

Pre-cut and Store Properly

If stored properly in an airtight glass Tupperware or CorningWare container, fresh pre-cut produce will not spoil and oxidize very quickly and most of the food's nutrients should also be preserved. Planning ahead can actually save a great deal of time later on, per this example. Let's say you come home late from work and you want to prepare a quick and easy meal. Envision this scenario: you planned ahead by cleaning, cutting, and bagging salad greens after you came home from the grocery store earlier in the week, you cooked enough rice for the entire week's worth of recipes, and you marinated some fish or poultry in the refrigerator before you left for work in the morning. Following the simple recipes in this book, it's very easy to put together pre-cut, pre-stored ingredients—cooking takes much less time, less heat, and less effort on your part. A quick, healthy, tasty meal can be ready in just minutes!

Simple, Easy Ways to Prepare Food for Longevity

Careful food preparation is the key to successfully eating to *thrive*. When it comes to preparing healthy meals, I like to keep the process simple and easy, which means planning and preparing ahead of time. Before making a big shopping trip, I spend a little time planning menus for the week and creating a detailed list of necessary items. When I come home from shopping, I clean and prepare the produce for the entire week. Following the week's menu, I dice fruits and/or vegetables and put them in a glass container with the other ingredients required for the same meal. I also make small, easy-to-carry bunches of produce for snacks and smaller meals. These time-saving steps make it easy to stick to your menu when you come home late from work, or when you're scanning the refrigerator for a snack.

Time-Saving Prep Methods

Everyone likes to save valuable time and energy! These tricks can help you save a little time and a lot of nutrients in your cooking techniques.

- Reserve your cooking water. If you cook kale in water, the same cooking water can be used as vegetable broth the next time you make rice, adding intense flavor and valuable nutrients.
- Make stocks and sauces in bulk and freeze them in ice-cube trays. Toss a couple cubes of frozen stock or sauce in various recipes for added flavor the next time you are cooking vegetables, grains, or meat.
- Make large batches of soups and sauces and freeze them in one-meal portions for later use. Frozen soups make excellent lunches and frozen sauces are helpful additions to quick dinner recipes.
- Soak beans overnight. This practice will save you a lot of time over the stove and will also save you from the potential hazards of canned food.
- Invest in a slow cooker or crockpot. Slow cookers help you easily plan ahead and make large portions of stews, beans, cereals, or grains for the entire week or for a large dinner party.
- Use your refrigerator and freezer to your advantage. I usually prepare enough cereal grains and beans for the week, and then immediately put half of the prepared food in the refrigerator and the other half in the freezer. By midweek, I have eaten the refrigerator portion, and then I move the freezer portion to the refrigerator to finish out the week. Using the refrigerator and freezer effectively can give your bulk-cooked meals a longer life span.

SPICE FOR LIFE

*"The art of healing comes from nature, not from the physician.
Therefore the physician must start from nature, with an open mind."*

—PARACELSUS

Dr. Mao's Longevity Spice Blends

Wouldn't it be great if you could simultaneously enrich the flavor of a dish while also improving its health benefits? Herbs and spices do just that! My spice blends will help support your health while they make your meals delicious! The ten spice combinations that appear below are meant to help with the ten conditions I most commonly see among my patients at the Tao of Wellness.

You will notice that these ten spice blends show up in various recipes that come later in this book. You are welcome to adjust and use other spice blends, according to your tastes and needs. In fact, if you are looking for a way to cut back on salt, you can experiment with replacing the salt that is called for in any given recipe with one of these spice blends instead.

HOW TO MAKE YOUR OWN SPICE BLENDS

You don't need to measure these out perfectly, but try to use equal amounts of each spice in its dried and ground forms. The consistency of the finished spice blend should be a powder. Any airtight glass jar stored in a dark, cool place will protect the volatile oils in these spice blends for between six months and a year.

The best time to add these spices to your meals is one minute before taking your food off the flame. Simply put in a teaspoon of the spice blend, stir, turn off the heat, and enjoy! These spice blends also work well for marinating proteins.

If collecting and grinding all these spices yourself isn't possible, you have the practical option of purchasing these ten spice blends, which have been carefully mixed at the Tao of Wellness, and are available on the Ask Dr. Mao website.

The herb blends that follow are meant to support your health, but you should not treat them as a cure-all or a replacement for medication. Some herbal supplements may interact with drug medications. As your health strategies change and evolve, never stop taking prescription medications without first speaking to your physician.

HEART SPICE BLEND

The herbs and spices in this spice blend are an all-around heart support, helpful for heart disease, high cholesterol, high blood pressure, pre-diabetes conditions, and diabetes.

- ground cinnamon
- fennel seed
- ground cloves
- ground star anise
- ground white pepper
- dried parsley
- ground ginger
- cayenne pepper
- turmeric

IMMUNITY SPICE BLEND

This blend will boost the strength of your immune system and also give you some support for cancer prevention.

- dried oregano
- dried cilantro
- garlic powder
- onion powder
- ground star anise
- dried basil
- dried thyme

ANTI-INFLAMMATORY SPICE BLEND

This spice blend helps combat inflammation, making it very helpful for arthritis support and muscle pain.

- dried basil
- cracked black pepper
- ground cinnamon
- chili powder
- ground cloves
- curry powder
- fennel seed
- dried marjoram
- ground nutmeg
- dried oregano
- dried rosemary
- dried sage
- dried tarragon
- dried thyme

METABOLISM SPICE BLEND

The herbs and spices in this blend help increase your energy level and boost the function of your metabolism, making it good for healthy weight management. This blend can be helpful for insulin resistance and pre-diabetes care.

- red chili pepper
- cayenne pepper
- dried seaweed
- dried kelp
- ground cumin seed
- ground mustard seed
- ground cinnamon
- garlic powder

CLEANSING SPICE BLEND

If you are looking to detoxify and cleanse your body, this spice blend will support you!

- turmeric
- ground ginger
- dried parsley
- dried rosemary
- cayenne pepper
- fenugreek
- fennel seed

DIGESTION SPICE/HERB BLEND

Without proper digestion, your body isn't able to absorb the nutrients from the healthy food you are eating. This blend supports healthy digestion, helping ensure regularity, absorb nutrients, and relieve heartburn, gas, and bloating.

- ground ginger
- dried peppermint
- turmeric
- ground cardamom
- ground star anise
- dried basil
- bay leaves
- dried dill
- fennel seed
- ground coriander
- dried oregano
- dried rosemary

BRAIN & VISION

A simple blend, the three herbs in this spice blend will enhance your cognitive function and eyesight.

- dried rosemary
- dried sage
- dried mint
- turmeric
- ground cinnamon
- ground cloves
- garlic powder

SKIN BEAUTY SPICE/HERB BLEND

From the ancient empresses of China, combined with Western research, this blend will support a youthful appearance, benefiting your skin, nails, and hair.

- turmeric
- dried rosemary
- dried sage
- dried basil
- dried and ground neem leaves
- dried parsley
- dried thyme
- dried oregano
- dried mint
- dried chives
- ground cinnamon

GOOD MOOD SPICE BLEND

This blend helps restore your happiness and is also helpful for alleviating stress.

- lavender
- dried and crushed rose
- dried sage
- chili powder
- ground saffron
- ground cardamom
- dried rosemary

SEXUAL HEALTH SPICE BLEND

Hormonal and sexual support for both women and men is supported by this blend.

- ground coriander
- ground ginger
- cayenne pepper
- ground cloves
- turmeric
- curry powder
- chili powder
- fenugreek
- fennel seed
- garlic powder
- ground cardamom
- ground nutmeg
- dried basil

MENUS FOR HEALING

"Those who take medicine and neglect their diet waste the skill of the physician." —CHINESE PROVERB

In traditional Chinese medicine, doctors focus on supporting the body so that it is strong enough to ward off and kill pathogens. The body can heal itself if given the proper chance, but sometimes we need to give the body a little help through nutritional measures or healing herbs.

The spice blends you just learned about are one way to support your health. The menus in this section build on that idea and take it to the next level. I selected these four menus in particular, because I believe they address the biggest threats to your longevity and quality of life: cardiovascular disease, stroke, cancer, diabetes, and inflammatory disorders. That said, you can easily create your own menus for the other condition categories, such as Brain & Vision or Cleansing. This section will give you a good idea of how to tailor a menu to suit your personal needs.

You will notice that the menus follow the concept of five meals a day. Your body functions best when fed at regular intervals, so try to eat your meals at these times:

- Breakfast should be eaten between 6:00 and 9:00 a.m.
- A mid-morning snack can come between 10:30 and 11:00 a.m.
- Lunch should be between 12:00 and 1:30 p.m.
- A mid-afternoon snack can come between 3:00 and 4:00 p.m.
- Dinner should come between 6:00 and 7:30 p.m.

Heart Menu

This menu is an all-around cardiovascular support, helpful for heart disease, high cholesterol, high blood pressure, pre-diabetes conditions, and diabetes. If you are at high risk for heart disease or it runs in your family, consider adopting this weekly menu for the ultimate healthy heart. If you are vegetarian, swap out the fish recipes with a vegetarian heart health option of your choice, and make sure you are getting enough omega-3s through high quality flaxseed oil or an omega-3 supplement. If you find yourself unprepared for a meal out, pick up the heart-supportive Middle Eastern dish tabouleh, which is high in fiber and vegetables.

DAY 1

Breakfast: Dr. Mao's Hot Herbal Cereal, pg. 77; *make full recipe, enough for 4 days*

Midmorning: 1 apple with 1 tablespoon of nut butter

Lunch: Salmon Leek Salad with Ginger-Miso Dressing, pg. 114

Afternoon: Soy Yogurt Dip with Carrots, Jicama, and Cucumber Sticks, pg. 163

Dinner: Vegetarian Hot and Sour Soup, pg. 89, with cooked brown rice; *make full recipe, enough for next-day lunch*

DAY 2

Breakfast: Dr. Mao's Hot Herbal Cereal, pg. 77

Midmorning: Anti-Aging Brain Mix, pg. 159

Lunch: Vegetarian Hot and Sour Soup, pg. 89

Afternoon: Soy Yogurt Dip with Carrots, Jicama, and Cucumber Sticks, pg. 163

Dinner: Stuffed Sardines with Pesto, pg. 142 (or Curry Vegetables with Brown Rice, pg. 133)

DAY 3

Breakfast: Dr. Mao's Hot Herbal Cereal, pg. 77, blended with Vegan Milk, pg. 62, with ¼ cup berries

Midmorning: ¼ cup mixed nuts and seeds

Lunch: Edamame, Seaweed and Tofu Salad, pg. 112

Afternoon: 1 apple with 1 tablespoon of nut butter

Dinner: Millet Pilaf, pg. 131; *make full recipe, save enough for next-day lunch*

DAY 4

Breakfast: Dr. Mao's Hot Herbal Cereal, pg. 77

Midmorning: ½ cup edamame

Lunch: Millet Pilaf, pg. 131

Afternoon: Black Bean Hummus, pg. 160, with cucumbers and carrots

Dinner: Creamy Sweet Potato Soup, pg. 95; *make full recipe, enough for next-day lunch*

DAY 5

Breakfast: Avocado, Flax, and Coconut Smoothie, pg. 67

Midmorning: Berrylicious and Delicious!, pg. 169

Lunch: Creamy Sweet Potato Soup, pg. 95

Afternoon: Black Bean Hummus, pg. 160, with celery sticks

Dinner: Salmon Leek Salad with Ginger-Miso Dressing, pg. 114, with side of Brown Rice with Pine Nuts, pg. 125

DAY 6

Breakfast: Muesli Parfait, pg. 73

Midmorning: 1 apple with 1 tablespoon of nut butter

Lunch: Brown Rice with Pine Nuts, pg. 125

Afternoon: Edamame Hummus, pg. 162, with seaweed chips

Dinner: Almond and Veggie Stir-Fry, pg. 124; *make full recipe, enough for next-day lunch*

DAY 7

Breakfast: Eggless Tofu Scramble, pg. 80

Midmorning: Edamame Hummus, pg. 162, with celery sticks

Lunch: Almond and Veggie Stir-Fry, pg. 124

Afternoon: Avocado, Flax, and Coconut Smoothie, pg. 67

Dinner: Baked Salmon with Lemon and Mango Salsa, pg. 141

Immunity Menu

This menu boosts the strength of your immune system, which is very helpful during cold and flu season, and it also gives you some support for cancer prevention. If you're one of those people who has a cold every few weeks, you may want to consider adopting this weekly menu. If your schedule doesn't allow a lot of time for food preparation, take a day off to prepare soups ahead of time and freeze in single-sized portions. A great immunity-boosting snack is make-your-own pickles. Simply cut up cruciferous vegatables (broccoli, cauliflower, Brussels sprouts, etc.) and garlic, put in a jar filled ½ inch from the top with rice vinegar, and let this pickle in your refrigerator for about a week. Instant snack!

DAY 1

Breakfast: Dr. Mao's Hot Herbal Cereal, pg. 77; *make full recipe, enough for 4 days*

Midmorning: Roast cauliflower, broccoli, and Brussels sprouts, following Braised Chicory with Red Wine Vinegar recipe, pg. 120; *make enough for 4 snack servings*

Lunch: Brown Rice with Pine Nuts, pg. 125, with roasted cauliflower, broccoli, and Brussels sprouts

Afternoon: Guacamole with Kale Chips, pg. 164

Dinner: Immunity-Boosting Borscht with Porcini Mushrooms, pg. 91; *make full recipe, save enough for next-day lunch*

DAY 2

Breakfast: Dr. Mao's Hot Herbal Cereal, pg. 77, with ¼ cup berries

Midmorning: Guacamole with Kale Chips, pg. 164

Lunch: Immunity-Boosting Borscht with Porcini Mushrooms, pg. 91

Afternoon: Energy Smoothie, pg. 61

Dinner: Broccoli Stir-Fry with Yam Noodles, pg. 123

DAY 3

Breakfast: Dr. Mao's Hot Herbal Cereal, pg. 77, with ¼ cup berries

Midmorning: Roasted cauliflower, broccoli, and Brussels sprouts

Lunch: Orange Fruit Salad with Maple-Glazed Ginger Pecans, pg. 105

Afternoon: Dried mushroom snacks, found in local health food stores

Dinner: Miso-Glazed Sole with Swiss Chard, pg. 148 (or Roasted Chestnuts and Wood Ear Mushrooms with Brown Rice, pg. 129, if vegetarian)

DAY 4

Breakfast: Dr. Mao's Hot Herbal Cereal, pg. 77, with ¼ cup berries

Midmorning: Energy Smoothie, pg. 61

Lunch: Brown Rice with Pine Nuts, pg. 125, with sautéed mushrooms

Afternoon: Pickled vegetables *(see directions in Immunity Menu introduction)*

Dinner: Immunity-Boosting Cream of Mushroom and Cauliflower Soup, pg. 94; *make full recipe, save enough for next-day lunch*

DAY 5

Breakfast: Egg White Scramble with Chard and Porcini Mushrooms, pg. 78

Midmorning: Anti-Aging Brain Mix, pg. 159

Lunch: Immunity-Boosting Cream of Mushroom and Cauliflower Soup, pg. 94

Afternoon: Pickled vegetables *(see directions in Immunity Menu introduction)*

Dinner: Zesty Halibut in Soy-Ginger Dressing, pg. 144 (or Stuffed Pumpkin, pg. 128, if vegetarian)

Breakfast: Energy Smoothie, pg. 61

Midmorning: Anti-Aging Brain Mix, pg. 159

Lunch: Orange Fruit Salad with Maple-Glazed Ginger Pecans, pg. 105

Afternoon: Guacamole with Kale Chips, pg. 164

Dinner: Immunity Soup, pg. 92; *make full recipe, save enough for next-day lunch*

Breakfast: Egg White Scramble with Chard and Porcini Mushrooms, pg. 78

Midmorning: Dried mushroom snacks, found in local health-food stores

Lunch: Immunity Soup, pg. 92, with millet

Afternoon: Pickled vegetables *(see directions in Immunity Menu introduction)*

Dinner: Broccoli Stir-Fry with Yam Noodles, pg. 123

Anti-Inflammation Menu

This menu helps combat inflammation, which is very helpful for arthritis support, muscle pain, and other inflammatory conditions. Consider trying this weekly menu if you have a pulled muscle, experience arthritis pain, or have a condition like tennis elbow or carpal tunnel syndrome. Leave any nightshade vegetables out of these recipes, including tomatoes, eggplant, and bell peppers, as these can make inflammatory pain worse. Also, make sure you are taking a daily dose of fish oil or flaxseed oil to help reduce inflammation.

Breakfast: Cool the Fire Tropical Smoothie, pg. 69

Midmorning: Baked Sweet Potato Chips with Pumpkin Seeds, pg. 166

Lunch: Mango-Avocado Salad, pg. 111

Afternoon: White Grape Lemonade, pg. 60

Dinner: Curry Vegetable with Brown Rice, pg. 133; *make full recipe, save enough for next-day lunch*

Breakfast: Muesli Parfait, pg. 73

Midmorning: Cup of green tea, with ½ cup of red grapes

Lunch: Curry Vegetable with Brown Rice, pg. 133

Afternoon: Baked Sweet Potato Chips with Pumpkin Seeds, pg. 166

Dinner: Mint Pea Falafel, pg. 138 (leave out eggs if vegan)

DAY 3

Breakfast: Dr. Mao's Hot Herbal Cereal, pg. 77; *make full recipe, enough for 4 days*

Midmorning: Anti-Aging Brain Mix, pg. 159

Lunch: Cool and Crunchy Salad, pg. 108

Afternoon: White Grape Lemonade, pg. 60, and ¼ cup sliced pineapple

Dinner: Spring Soup, pg. 96; *make full recipe, save enough for next-day lunch*

DAY 4

Breakfast: Dr. Mao's Hot Herbal Cereal, pg. 77

Midmorning: ¼ cup sliced pineapple

Lunch: Spring Soup, pg. 96

Afternoon: Cup of green tea, with ¼ cup berries

Dinner: ½ recipe of Cool and Crunchy Salad, pg. 108, with Saffron Ginger Fish Soup, pg. 102 (or Immunity Soup, pg. 92, if vegetarian); *make full recipe, save enough for next-day lunch*

DAY 5

Breakfast: Dr. Mao's Hot Herbal Cereal, pg. 77, with ¼ cup berries

Midmorning: Anti-Aging Brain Mix, pg. 159

Lunch: Saffron Ginger Fish Soup, pg. 102 (or Immunity Soup, pg. 92, if vegetarian)

Afternoon: Cool the Fire Tropical Smoothie, pg. 69

Dinner: Black Bass with Coriander, pg. 145 (or Vegetable Almond Pie, pg. 126, if vegetarian)

DAY 6

Breakfast: Dr. Mao's Hot Herbal Cereal, pg. 77, with ¼ cup Vegan Milk, pg. 62

Midmorning: Cool the Fire Tropical Smoothie, pg. 69

Lunch: Mango-Avocado Salad, pg. 111

Afternoon: Cup of green tea and 1 sliced kiwi

Dinner: Mint Pea Falafel, pg. 138 (leave out eggs if vegan); *make full recipe, save enough for next-day lunch*

Breakfast: Eggless Tofu Scramble, pg. 80
Midmorning: Cup of Vegan Milk, pg. 62, with ¼ cup berries
Lunch: Mint Pea Falafel, pg. 138 (leave out eggs if vegan)
Afternoon: Baked Sweet Potato Chips with Pumpkin Seeds, pg. 166
Dinner: Curry Vegetable with Brown Rice, pg. 133

Metabolism Menu

This menu helps increase your energy level and boosts the function of your metabolism, which is beneficial for healthy weight management. Implementing this weekly menu will help you lose weight in a healthy way—you'll feel great! This menu also offers support for insulin resistance and pre-diabetes care. You will notice that one of the main ingredients on this menu is seaweed—from the snacking nori seaweed strips you can pick up in health food stores to soaked wakame and cut-up kombu, there are plenty of ways to use seaweed in your cooking. Feel free to add more to the meals in this section.

DAY 1

Breakfast: Energy Smoothie, pg. 61
Midmorning: Avocado Hummus, pg. 161, with seaweed crackers
Lunch: Edamame, Seaweed and Tofu Salad, pg. 112
Afternoon: Anti-Aging Brain Mix, pg. 159
Dinner: Chicken Leek Soup with Dried Plums and Quinoa, pg. 99 (or Immunity Soup, pg. 92, if vegetarian); *make full recipe, save enough for next-day lunch*

DAY 2

Breakfast: Dr. Mao's Hot Herbal Cereal, pg. 77; *make full recipe, enough for 4 days*
Midmorning: seaweed strips
Lunch: Chicken Leek Soup with Dried Plums and Quinoa, pg. 99 (or Immunity Soup, pg. 92, if vegetarian)
Afternoon: Avocado Hummus, pg. 161, with seaweed crackers
Dinner: Millet Pilaf, pg. 131

DAY 3

Breakfast: Dr. Mao's Hot Herbal Cereal, pg. 77, with ¼ cup berries
Midmorning: Energy Smoothie, pg. 61

Lunch: Edamame, Seaweed and Tofu Salad, pg. 112

Afternoon: Anti-Aging Brain Mix, pg. 159

Dinner: Seaweed and Vegetable Medley, pg. 121; *make full recipe, save enough for next-day lunch*

DAY 4

Breakfast: Dr. Mao's Hot Herbal Cereal, pg. 77, with ¼ cup berries

Midmorning: Anti-Aging Brain Mix, pg. 159

Lunch: Seaweed and Vegetable Medley, pg. 121

Afternoon: ½ cup edamame

Dinner: Creamy Sweet Potato Soup, pg. 95, with side of millet; *make full recipe, save enough for next-day lunch*

DAY 5

Breakfast: Dr. Mao's Hot Herbal Cereal, pg. 77, with ¼ cup berries

Midmorning: Seaweed strips

Lunch: Creamy Sweet Potato Soup, pg. 95

Afternoon: Energy Smoothie, pg. 61

Dinner: Chicken Leek Soup with Dried Plums and Quinoa, pg.99 (or Spring Soup, pg. 96, if vegetarian); *make full recipe, save enough for next-day lunch*

DAY 6

Breakfast: Savory Oatmeal with Pine Nuts, Avocado, and Egg, pg.74 (or Eggless Tofu Scramble, pg. 80, if vegetarian)

Midmorning: Anti-Aging Brain Mix, pg. 159

Lunch: Chicken Leek Soup with Dried Plums and Quinoa, pg. 99 (or Spring Soup, pg. 96, if vegetarian)

Afternoon: Black Bean Hummus, pg. 160, with seaweed strips

Dinner: Sautéed King Prawns with Chestnut and Figs, pg. 151 (or Seaweed and Vegetable Medley, pg. 121, if vegetarian)

DAY 7

Breakfast: Energy Smoothie, pg. 61

Midmorning: Black Bean Hummus, pg. 160, with carrot and cucumber sticks

Lunch: Edamame, Seaweed and Tofu Salad, pg. 112

Afternoon: Anti-Aging Brain Mix, pg. 159

Dinner: Seaweed and Vegetable Medley, pg. 121

BEVERAGES

The beverages in this section come from all over the world, including longevity hot spots like the Hunza Valley and Vilcabamba, Ecuador. Be sure to make juice and smoothies fresh before drinking, as nutrients are lost the longer the juice sits out. Whether you drink one of the lemonades to cool down on a summer day or choose a smoothie for breakfast, you will reap the rewards of these nutritious drinks for years to come.

DR. MAO'S HONEY LEMONADE

BENEFITS: IMMUNITY + CLEANSING + DIGESTION + ANTI-AGING BEAUTY

My grandmother used to make this honey lemonade to cure everything, from stomachaches to heat exhaustion. This naturally sweet beverage is refreshing during the hot days of summer and helps protect you from infections in your gut, an event most common in very hot weather when your food is sitting out gathering bacteria. Honey is a natural antibacterial and the lemon's acidity helps inhibit bacteria, all good actions to have working for your digestive tract. Also, lemon is an alkalizer, which will further help steady the stomach.

SERVES 6 TO 8

1 cup freshly squeezed lemon juice
  (from about 8 large lemons)
½ to ¾ cup honey, to taste
8 to 9 cups water
1 lemon, thinly sliced, for serving

In a large pitcher, stir the lemon juice, ½ cup honey, and 8 cups of water together until the honey is completely dissolved. Taste and adjust the strength and sweetness with more honey and water, if needed. Stir in the lemon slices and refrigerate until very cold. Serve poured over ice.

Honey has long been known for its antibiotic properties and is much more nutritious than refined table sugar. As a folk remedy, honey has been taken for stomach ulcers and heartburn, and Western research indicates that it may stop the growth of *H. pylori*, the bacteria responsible for most gastric ulcers. The caffeic acid in honey may also prevent colon cancer. *Never give honey to a child under one year of age.*

WHITE GRAPE LEMONADE

BENEFITS: IMMUNITY + ANTI-INFLAMMATION + CLEANSING + DIGESTION

Here is another sweet treat for a hot day! In addition to the cooling and stomach soothing actions of lemon juice, white grapes offer a mild anti-inflammatory action, helpful for relieving inflammation within the body that over time, could trigger chronic illness, such as heart disease, stroke, cancer, diabetes, sleep disorders, Alzheimer's, and arthritis. While the benefits are particularly helpful in the summer, this lemonade is a pleasure to sip year-round.

SERVES 6 TO 8

1   cup freshly squeezed lemon juice (from about 8 large lemons)

½   to ¾ cup white grape juice concentrate, to taste

8   to 9 cups water

1   lemon, thinly sliced, for serving

In a large pitcher, stir the lemon juice, ½ cup grape juice concentrate, and 8 cups of water together until the concentrate is completely dissolved. Taste and adjust the strength and sweetness with more grape juice concentrate and water, if needed. Stir in the lemon slices and refrigerate until very cold. Serve poured over ice.

The high vitamin C content in **lemons** has been famous since New World exploration for its use in preventing scurvy. Vitamin C is one of the most powerful antioxidants, effective at controlling inflammatory conditions like arthritis, staving off cholesterol build-up, and supporting a healthy immune system. Lemons also contain limonoid, a phytonutrient that is thought to combat many types of cancer and possibly protect against cardiovascular disease.

ENERGY SMOOTHIE

BENEFITS: IMMUNITY + METABOLISM + BRAIN & VISION + SEXUAL HEALTH

This smoothie is fantastic for promoting energy and is packed with nutrition. The base for this high-protein, low-calorie beverage is antioxidant-rich blueberries and potassium-rich bananas mixed with almond milk, which not only adds flavor, but also essential fatty acids and calcium. If you opt to use the High Performance Powder and Five Elements Powder—which includes 44 potent Chinese herbs, chlorophyll, and fiber—you will be benefiting from over 50 Chinese herbs in there that are specifically meant to increase vital energy and longevity. While you could techni-cally mix the herbs together to make these two traditional Chinese herbal blends, it would be more practical to purchase them already blended by expert traditional Chinese medicine doctors. These are both available at www.AskDrMao.com.

SERVES 2

1½ cups almond milk
1   banana
½   cup fresh or frozen blueberries
½   cup plain coconut yogurt
2   tablespoons wildflower honey
2   tablespoons High Performance
     Powder
2   tablespoons Five Elements
     Powder

Put all of the ingredients into a blender and blend until smooth. Divide between two glasses and serve immediately.

Of all fruits, **blueberries** have one of the highest levels of antioxidant activity, helping to reduce the risk of certain cancers and bringing anti-aging benefits. Blueberries have neuroprotective proper-ties that can delay the onset of age-related memory loss by shielding brain cells from damage by chemicals, plaque, or trauma. They have also been shown to lower blood cholesterol and lipid levels. They are high in manganese and vitamin K, and have a very low glycemic load, making them an ideal fruit for diabetics. All this, and delicious, too!

VEGAN MILK

BENEFITS OF HEMP MILK: HEART + DIGESTION + BRAIN & VISION + ANTI-AGING BEAUTY

BENEFITS OF ALMOND MILK: HEART + ANTI-INFLAMMATION + BRAIN & VISION + ANTI-AGING BEAUTY

I am not personally a fan of dairy foods. Luckily, this recipe gives you so many delicious, nutritious variations on vegan milk that you will not even miss cow's milk! Almond milk is one of my favorites, as it has the best nutritional profile versus animal milk. Another highly nutritious option is hemp milk, a food recipe from centenarians in Bama, China, who credit their hemp food products for their health and longevity. Don't worry, there are absolutely no psychedelic qualities in hemp seeds! On the contrary, these seeds are full of perfectly balanced fatty acids, helpful for reducing inflammation and at the same time increasing circulation. So go ahead and make your own protein-rich, nutritious version.

SERVES 4

1 cup nuts or seeds, or beans or legumes of your choice
6 cups water
½ teaspoon vanilla or almond extract
2 tablespoons sweetener (honey, maple syrup, stevia powder, ground dates, or raisin puree)
   Pinch of ground cinnamon or ground cardamom

TO MAKE MILK FROM NUTS OR SEEDS:

1. Soak the raw nuts or seeds for at least 4 hours in fresh, cold water. Drain the nuts or seeds and transfer them to a blender. Pour in 2 cups of fresh water and blend on high speed until smooth. Pour the mixture through a fine mesh strainer set over a pitcher, pressing on the solids. Put the solids back into the blender jar, add another 2 cups of fresh water, and blend again on high until smooth. Strain the mixture again, adding to the liquid in the pitcher. Repeat the process one more time.

2. Combining all of the strained "milk," there should be a total of 6 cups. Rinse out the blender and put about 1 cup of the liquid back in the blender with the vanilla, sweetener of your choice, and cinnamon or cardamom. Blend until well combined and stir into the unseasoned milk. Store in the refrigerator and use within a few days.

I have made **plant milk** from just about everything: garbanzo beans, black beans, sesame seeds, peanuts, cashews—you name it. If you are willing to experiment, it is worth the effort, but you have to be open to a different look and taste. Peanuts make a delicious peanut-butter-flavored milk that is rich in protein, with good portions of fatty acids and calcium. Black bean milk, also very nutritious, looks a little intimidating with its grayish-beige hue. Experiment, and have fun!

TO MAKE MILK FROM BEANS OR LEGUMES:

1. Soak the beans or legumes overnight in fresh, cold water for 8 hours.

2. Line a fine mesh strainer with cheesecloth and drain the beans or legumes, discarding the liquid, and rinse them well under cold running water. Transfer the beans and any fiber residue in the cheesecloth to a blender and add 2 cups of fresh water. Blend on high speed until smooth. Pour the mixture through a fine mesh strainer set over a pitcher, pressing on the solids. Put the solids back into the blender, add another 2 cups of fresh water, and blend again on high until smooth. Strain the mixture again, adding to the liquid in the pitcher. Repeat the process one more time.

3. Pour the strained liquid into a saucepan over medium heat and bring to a boil. Reduce the heat to low and simmer the liquid for 30 minutes; let stand until cool.

4. Rinse out the blender and put about 1 cup of the liquid back in the blender with the vanilla, sweetener of your choice, and cinnamon or cardamom. Blend until well combined and stir into the unseasoned milk. Store in the refrigerator and use within a few days.

Hemp seeds are full of perfectly balanced fatty acids, helpful for reducing inflammation and at the same time increasing circulation. Hemp seeds are also rich in nutrients, including vitamin E and other immune-boosting compounds. Hemp milk contains ten essential amino acids and for some is easier to digest than cow's milk.

HUNZA BRAIN TONIC

BENEFITS: BRAIN & VISION + GOOD MOOD

This blended drink is based on a recipe by a centenarian I met from the Hunza Valley, an area in modern-day Pakistan that is famed for its long-living citizens. Many apricot trees grow in this region, which explains apricot's prominence in this recipe. Apricots are rich in antioxidant carotenoids, which impart the fruit with its orangey color and help protect against heart disease and cancer. The egg yolk has lecithin, which has been found to help brain function and protect against some cancers. Kelp powder can be found in most health-food stores or specialty herb and supplement stores.

SERVES 1

½ cup chopped fresh apricots, or chopped dried apricots soaked in hot water and drained
1   teaspoon fresh lemon juice
½ teaspoon kelp powder
1   large organic egg yolk
1   cup cold soy or goat milk

Put the apricots, lemon juice, kelp powder, egg yolk, and milk into a blender and puree until smooth. Transfer to a glass and drink immediately.

Rich in vitamin A, C, and dietary fiber, **apricots** are one of the staple foods of the famously long-lived centenarians in the Hunza Valley. Apricots are also incredibly high in carotenoids, antioxidants that give them their characteristic orangey-yellow coloring and help prevent heart disease, reduce "bad cholesterol" levels, and protect against cancer. Meanwhile, vitamin A promotes good vision, and due to their high fiber-to-volume ratio, dried apricots are sometimes used to relieve constipation.

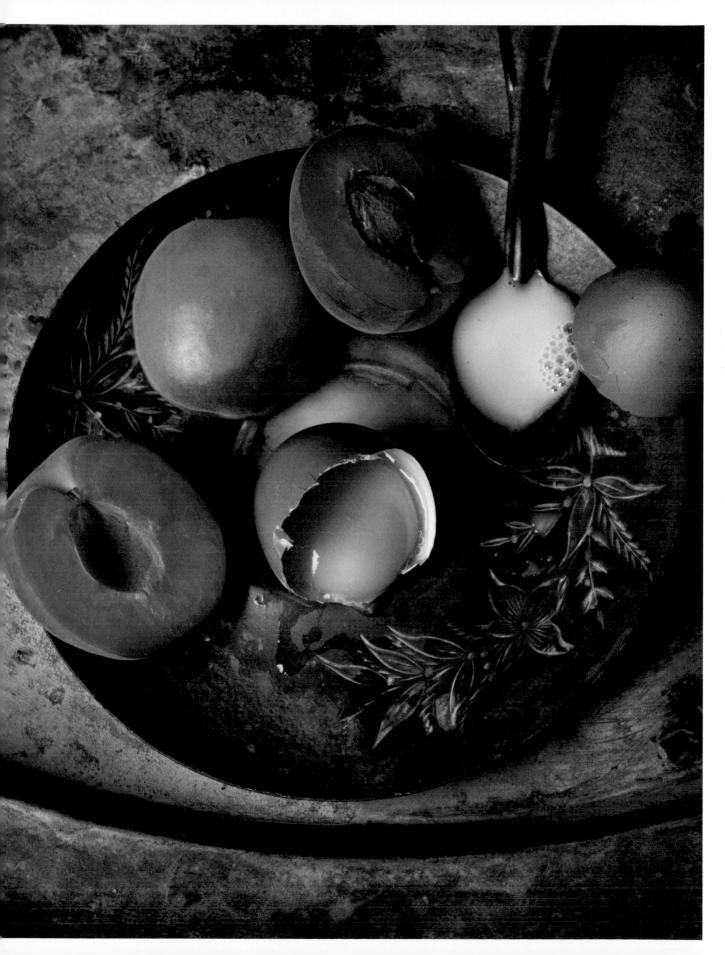

AVOCADO-GOJI BERRY SMOOTHIE

BENEFITS: ANTI-INFLAMMATION + BRAIN & VISION + ANTI-AGING BEAUTY

Avocado smoothies are popular in South America and Asia. This adaptation is based on a recipe from the Vilcabamba Valley in the southern region of Ecuador, a famous longevity spot. They don't have goji berries in this region, but I added them here so that you could benefit from their amazing antioxidant actions. Goji berries have among the highest levels of carotenoid antioxidants known. Avocados, meanwhile, have one of the highest instances of glutathione, which is one of the most potent antioxidants in nature. Together, they form a delicious anti-aging elixir.

SERVES 2

1   avocado, peeled and pitted
¾   cup hemp milk
¾   cup cranberry juice
¼   cup dried goji berries, soaked for
     1 hour in water and drained

Put all of the ingredients into a blender and blend until smooth. Divide between two glasses and serve immediately.

Avocados come up frequently in these recipes, and that is because they are incredibly healthy. Rich in heart-healthy monounsaturated fat, avocados are packed with the powerful antioxidant glutathione. This naturally occurring compound regulates immune cells, protects against cancer, and assists in detoxification. A deficiency in glutathione can play a part in diabetes, liver disease, heart disease, low sperm count, and premature aging. Avocados are also a source of L-cysteine, which may boost immunity, protect you from heart disease, build muscle, and encourage healthy hair and nail growth.

AVOCADO, FLAX, AND COCONUT SMOOTHIE

BENEFITS: HEART + ANTI-INFLAMMATION + DIGESTION + BRAIN & VISION + ANTI-AGING BEAUTY

Hailing from South America, this recipe features a trio of essential fatty acid powerhouses: avocados, flax, and coconut milk. These ingredients have anti-inflammatory properties and are important for brain health and hormonal health.

SERVES 2

2   cups loosely packed spinach
1½ cups coconut milk
1   avocado, peeled and pitted
½   cucumber, coarsely chopped
1   lemon, peeled and seeds removed
1   tablespoon ground flaxseeds
1   tablespoon sesame tahini
1   teaspoon maple syrup

Put all of the ingredients into a blender and blend until smooth. Divide between two glasses and serve immediately.

Flaxseeds have gained fame in the nutrition spotlight for their rich content of alpha linolenic acid (ALA), a plant-based omega-3 fatty acid. Flaxseeds are an excellent vegetarian source of heart-healthy omegas that contain anti-inflammatory properties. They also contain lignans, hormone-like compounds that may protect women against breast cancer and reduce the incidence of hot flashes that come with menopause. Make sure to always grind the seeds before eating so that it is easier for your body to assimilate the nutrients.

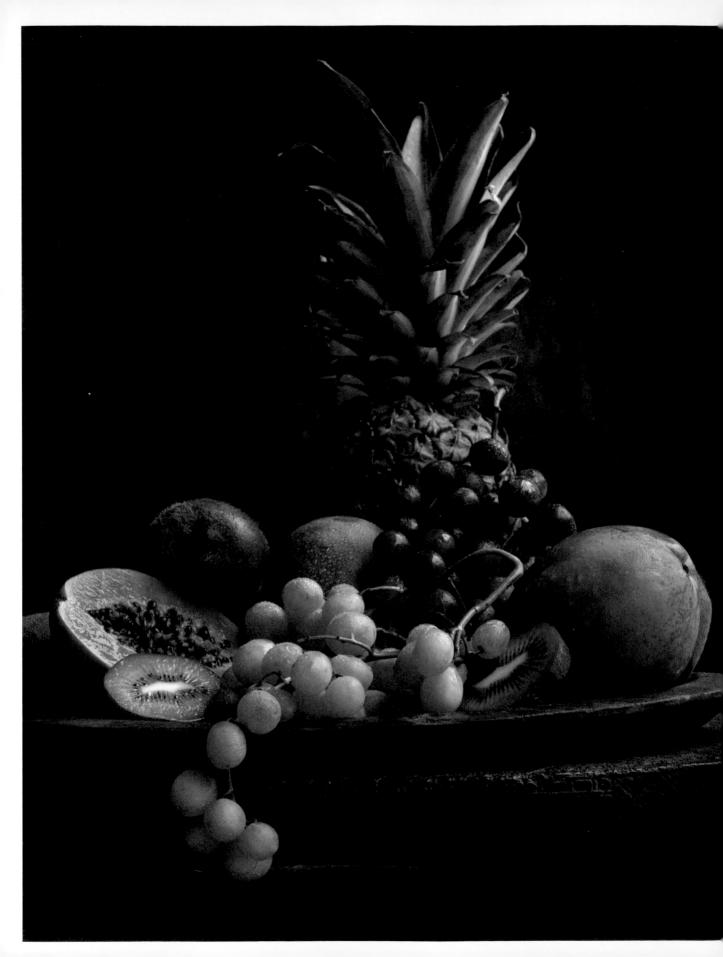

COOL THE FIRE TROPICAL SMOOTHIE

BENEFITS: HEART + IMMUNITY + ANTI-INFLAMMATION + METABOLISM + DIGESTION

This recipe came from a region in Southern China called Hainan Island, a resort island that is also famous for its population of centenarians. The Hainan people drink this year-round to help with digestion. Tropical fruits are filled with enzymes: the pineapple is rich in bromelain and the papaya contains papain, both natural anti-inflammatory substances, good for arthritis relief, diabetes prevention, and heart disease protection.

SERVES 4

½ fresh pineapple, peeled, cored, and coarsely chopped

2 kiwi, peeled and coarsely chopped

1 small papaya, peeled, seeded, and coarsely chopped

1 cup seedless grapes

1 cup unsweetened cherry juice

2 heaping tablespoons hemp powder

1 tablespoon flaxseed oil

2 cups almond milk, chilled

Put all of the ingredients into a blender and blend until smooth. Divide among four glasses and serve immediately.

Papayas are probably most famous for their protein-digesting enzymes, like chymopapain and papain. These enzymes calm inflammatory conditions, such as arthritis and asthma, promote strong digestion, and keep the intestines clean. Papaya's rich content of vitamins A, C, and E helps protect vision, bolster the immune system, and prevent cholesterol from oxidizing and clogging arteries, a risk factor for stroke and heart attack.

Pineapples contain bromelain, a mixture of protein-digesting enzymes, which contain active substances that help reduce inflammation and aid in digestion. Bromelain is linked with anti-inflammatory, anti-coagulant, and anti-cancer properties. Like papayas, pineapples boast high levels of vitamins A, C, and E.

INTERNAL CLEANSE TEA

BENEFITS: CLEANSING

This caffeine-free herbal tea blend, based on a classic liver-nourishing formula by the ancient Taoist masters of China, helps rid the body of harmful chemicals and toxins that we encounter in everyday life. Some of these ingredients will take a little research to find, but you should have success at specialty herb shops, some Asian markets, some health-food stores, and online. You can also purchase this tea online on the Ask Dr. Mao site.

SERVES 8

1   tablespoon white mulberry leaves
1   tablespoon dried mint
1   tablespoon sweetleaf leaves
1   tablespoon chrysanthemum
    flowers
1   tablespoon hawthorn fruit
1   tablespoon cassia tora seeds
1   tablespoon licorice root
1   tablespoon cocklebur fruit

Grind and mix the herbs together and store in a glass jar with a lid. Steep 1 tablespoon of the herbal tea blend for 5 minutes in boiled water. Drink 3 times a day for extra cleansing results.

Chrysanthemum flower is traditionally used to cleanse the liver, neutralize toxins, brighten vision, and cool one down in the heat of summer. It has been found that chrysanthemum lowers blood pressure and cholesterol and balances blood sugar.

EMOTIONAL TRANQUILITY TEA

BENEFITS: GOOD MOOD + SLEEP

Another caffeine-free herbal blend, this tea is based on a traditional Chinese medical formula for settling the mind and soothing the emotions—without causing drowsiness. This blend is especially helpful for relieving stress and insomnia. Look for these herbs at specialty herb shops, Asian markets, health-food stores, and online. You can also purchase this tea on the Ask Dr. Mao site.

SERVES 12

1 tablespoon chamomile flower
1 tablespoon licorice root
1 tablespoon lily bulb
1 tablespoon Chinese senega root
1 tablespoon bamboo shavings
1 tablespoon light wheat grain
1 tablespoon zizyphus seed
1 tablespoon China root
1 tablespoon curcuma root
1 tablespoon tientsin millet
1 tablespoon mimosa tree bark
1 tablespoon anise
1 tablespoon sweetleaf leaves

Grind and mix the herbs together and store in a glass jar with a lid. Steep 1 tablespoon of the herbal tea blend for 5 minutes in boiled water. Drink 3 times a day to promote restful sleep and allay anxiety.

Native to Eastern Europe, but now found almost all over the world, **chamomile flower** is a very well known herb for remedying sleep issues. It is part of the sunflower family, but this daisy-like flower is much smaller than its familiar cousin. Chamomile is also an excellent herb for settling the stomach. It also soothes the nervous system and relaxes the muscles, making it a perfect choice for the evening, an hour before bed.

BREAKFASTS

Start the day right with a breakfast that gives you the energy you need to function strong all day long! As it turns out, breakfast may really be the most important meal of the day owing to the fact that your body processes foods differently at different times of day. Studies have shown that when you eat your daily protein and fat at breakfast, you tend to have more energy and be less prone to weight gain. These recipes offer just that, with their balanced contributions of protein and healthy fats in each meal.

Even though this is the designated breakfast section of the book, it doesn't mean you can't start your day with a smoothie from the beverage section or a bowl of brown rice from the small dishes section! In fact, I had a very healthy patient in her eighties who used to begin her day with a bowl of seaweed miso soup, a common breakfast in Japan. So choose what is most appealing to you—just make sure you eat your breakfast before 9:00 a.m. to take advantage of your body's natural timing.

MUESLI PARFAIT

BENEFITS: HEART + ANTI-INFLAMMATION + CLEANSING + DIGESTION

A patient from Switzerland shared this recipe that her whole family has been eating for several generations. The grandparents and great-grandparents all lived to be in their nineties, and her parents, in their eighties, still hike in the Alps! It is easy to see the longevity-promoting characteristics of this recipe: hearty, complex whole grains are combined with the protein of nuts and seeds and the probiotics of cultured yogurt. I changed her original recipe a little by replacing the whole-milk yogurt with non-dairy yogurt, to take into account that dairy products in America are nowhere near as nutritious as those of Europe. I have a lot to say on the subject of dairy, which you can read on page 11.

SERVES 4

2   cups gluten-free rolled oats
½   cup blanched, sliced almonds
½   cup pecan halves
½   cup walnut halves
¼   cup sunflower seeds
1   cup fresh blueberries
½   cup chopped fresh figs (about 4 whole)
½   cup chopped fresh apricots (about 4 whole)
½   cup chopped fresh strawberries (about 8 large whole)
2   cups plain, live-culture soy or coconut yogurt

1. In a medium bowl, stir the oats, almonds, pecans, walnuts, and sunflower seeds together until combined. Add the blueberries, figs, apricots, and strawberries and gently mix until combined.

2. Fill 4 parfait glasses one-third full with the nut/fruit mixture. Divide the yogurt among the glasses and spoon the remaining muesli evenly over the top of the yogurt in each glass. Serve immediately.

A daily serving of **yogurt** is rich in probiotics, which increases your body's ability to protect you from infection. These live active cultures help stimulate cellular immunity, your immune system's first line of defense, which protects you from viruses, yeasts, parasites, and also helps prevent the development of cancer, so you can live a long and healthy life. I recommend soy or coconut yogurt, which is much easier to digest than cow's milk yogurt. If you insist on animal milk, I suggest goat's milk yogurt.

SAVORY OATMEAL WITH PINE NUTS, AVOCADO, AND EGG

BENEFITS: HEART + IMMUNITY + ANTI-INFLAMMATION + METABOLISM + DIGESTION

A healthy interpretation of the typical modern breakfast, this recipe really packs a nutritional punch. Instead of the rich and heavy usual breakfast suspects, like sausage, bacon, or fried eggs, this recipe features lighter, healthier foods that achieve a balance between protein, carbohydrates, and good fats. You get fiber from the oatmeal, protein from the eggs, and essential fatty acids from the pine nuts and avocado. You can still start the morning by eating like a king, but without the repercussions to your stomach and your health.

SERVES 1

1 tablespoon pine nuts
   Pinch of garlic powder
   Pinch of black pepper
   Pinch of dried chives
   Pinch of red chili flakes
½ cup organic, steel-cut oats
1 egg
¼ avocado, sliced, for garnish
1 small tomato, finely chopped, for garnish

1. Put the pine nuts in a small dry skillet over medium heat. Toast them briefly, swirling the pan. When they begin to brown lightly, add the garlic powder, pepper, chives, and chili flakes and stir constantly until the spices are fragrant and the pine nights are lightly browned. Remove promptly from the heat and set aside.

2. Bring 1½ cups of water to a boil and stir in the oats. Reduce the heat and simmer for 3 minutes. Crack the egg and stir it into the oats for about 30 seconds, or until the egg is cooked. Transfer the oats to a serving bowl. Sprinkle the toasted pine nut mixture over the top and garnish with slices of avocado and chopped tomato.

Steel-cut oats are whole grain groats that have been chopped into pieces. Rich in magnesium and fiber, oats can significantly lower the risk of cardiovascular disease, obesity, insulin resistance, and type 2 diabetes. Also, the saponins in oats increase production of natural "killer cells," enhancing the body's response to infection. Oats are the only cereal that contain the legume-like protein avenalin; in fact, oats have almost the same quality protein content as soy protein! While oats are technically gluten-free, they are often contaminated with gluten from other grains handled in close proximity. Look for packaging that specifies "gluten-free."

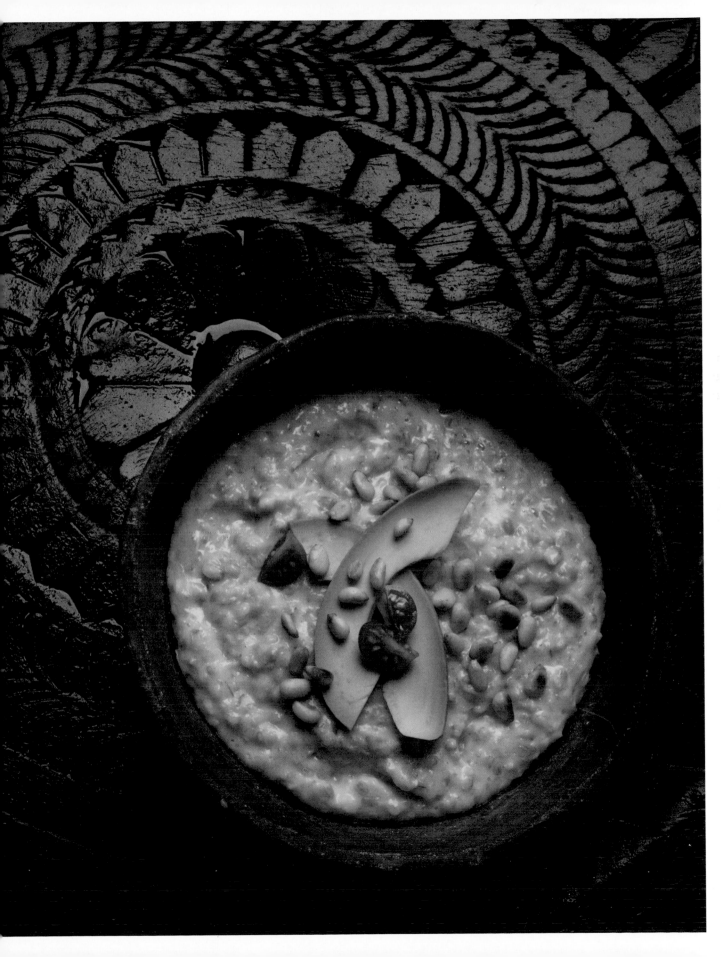

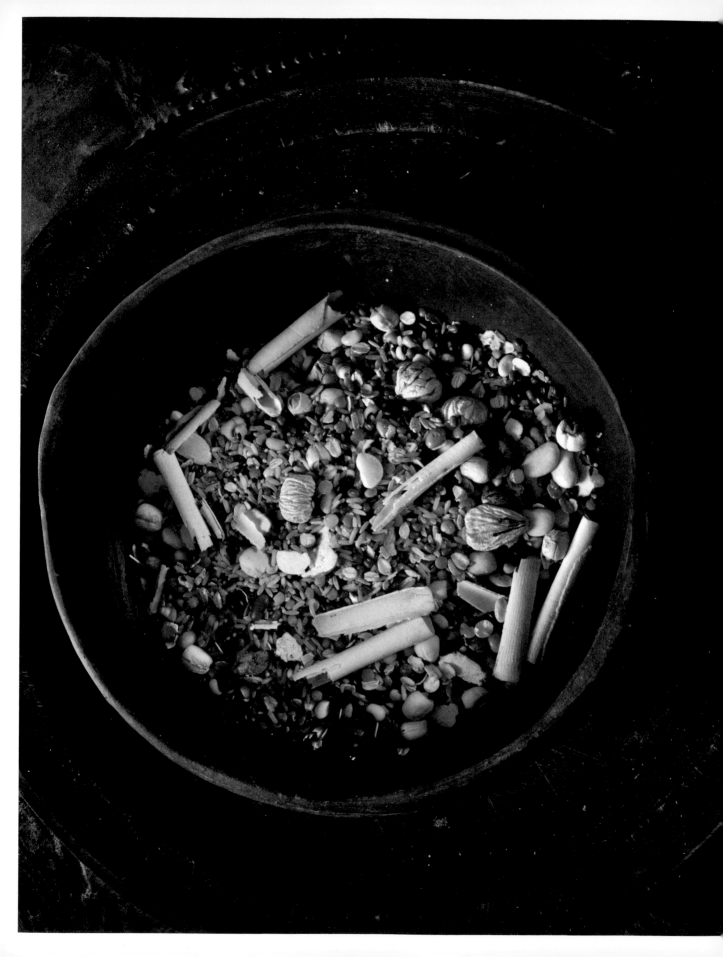

DR. MAO'S HOT HERBAL CEREAL

BENEFITS: HEART + IMMUNITY + ANTI-INFLAMMATION + METABOLISM + CLEANSING + DIGESTION + ANTI-AGING BEAUTY + GOOD MOOD

My family has been eating this herbal cereal for generations. One glance at this recipe, and you might think this is a practical joke—but I assure you, I personally eat this for breakfast every day. When else can you eat a variety of twenty-five foods in one meal? The wide array of herbs, nuts, seeds, whole grains, and legumes really make this a one-stop, complete-nutrition meal.

SERVES 4

GRAINS
¼ cup brown rice
¼ cup black rice
¼ cup gluten-free oats
¼ cup millet

NUTS AND SEEDS
⅓ cup peeled chestnuts
2 tablespoons sesame seeds

BEANS AND LEGUMES
¼ cup dried kidney beans
¼ cup dried adzuki beans
¼ cup dried pink beans
¼ cup dried white beans
¼ cup dried lima beans
¼ cup dried pinto beans
¼ cup dried black beans
¼ cup dried mung beans
¼ cup red lentils
¼ cup green lentils
¼ cup green split peas
¼ cup yellow split peas
¼ cup dried black-eyed peas

HERBS
¼ cup fox nut seeds
¼ cup loose dried wild yam root
¼ cup lotus seeds
¼ cup dried goji berries

8 cups filtered water
  Warm Almond Milk, pg. 62
  or soy milk, for serving
  Fresh berries, for serving
  Maple syrup, for serving, optional

1. Put all of the grains, nuts and seeds, beans and legumes, fox nut seeds, wild yam root, and lotus seeds into a large bowl and cover with water; soak overnight.

2. Drain the ingredients and transfer them to a large saucepan. Add the goji berries and water and bring to a boil. Reduce the heat to maintain a low simmer, partially cover, and cook, stirring frequently, until the beans and grains are soft but not mushy, 1 to 2 hours, depending on how soft you like the cereal.

3. To serve, ladle the cereal into bowls, pour a little warm milk over each bowl, and top with fresh berries and a dab of maple syrup, if you want it a little sweeter.

4. Store leftover cooled cereal in an airtight container in the refrigerator for up to 10 days.

NOTE: The cereal can also be made in a crockpot, no soaking necessary. Put all of the grains, nuts and seeds, beans and legumes, herbs, and the water into a slow cooker set on low. Cook for 8 hours or overnight until the dried beans are soft.

You can tweak the flavor of this herbal cereal. To make it sweet, add berries, chop up dates, or add a small amount of maple syrup or honey. To make it savory, add chopped onions. You can even add a spice mix tailored to your health concern. *Find out how to make your own spice blends on page 47 or you can purchase pre-mixed from the Ask Dr. Mao website.*

EGG WHITE SCRAMBLE WITH CHARD AND PORCINI MUSHROOMS

BENEFITS: HEART + IMMUNITY + DIGESTION

This is my variation on a recipe that comes from Sardinia. A patient of mine shared this recipe with me. It was a favorite of her grandmother, who lived to the ripe old age of 102. Her version used farm-fresh whole eggs from her own chickens; although this is a delicious and nutritious idea, most of us don't have chickens running around in our back yards! The featured ingredient, porcini mushrooms—and most mushrooms, for that matter—are high in fiber with virtually no fat, very helpful for lowering cholesterol and cleansing the intestinal tract. Meanwhile, the high-fiber chard also gives your heart health a boost with its minerals magnesium and potassium.

SERVES 2

2 teaspoons avocado oil
1 clove garlic, crushed
1 small bunch Swiss chard, finely chopped
8 fresh porcini mushrooms, chopped
6 large egg whites
   Sea salt and freshly ground black pepper
¼ red bell pepper, finely chopped, for garnish

1. Heat the oil in a large nonstick skillet over medium heat. Add the garlic and cook, stirring, until fragrant, about 1 minute. Add the chard and mushrooms and cook, stirring, until mushrooms are softened and chard is just limp, 3 to 4 minutes. Drain any excess liquid from the pan.

2. Reduce the heat to medium-low and pour in the egg whites. Cook, stirring gently, until just set, 1 to 2 minutes. Season with salt and pepper to taste and remove from the heat. Garnish with chopped red pepper and serve immediately.

The ancient Greeks and Romans celebrated **chard** for its many medicinal properties. So it's no surprise that it shows up in this recipe from Sardinia. High in fiber, chard is full of beneficial vitamins and nutrients. Chard's potassium and magnesium content helps prevent high blood pressure, the vitamin A and beta-carotene support vision health, and vitamin K and calcium maintain bone health. One cup of chard provides nearly one-fourth of your daily intake of iron, keeping your immune system healthy and helping your body produce energy. What a great green way to start your day!

BANANA BUCKWHEAT PANCAKES

BENEFITS: HEART + DIGESTION

Pancakes in a longevity cookbook? Absolutely, as long as the main ingredient is buckwheat! Buckwheat makes this Southern recipe quite healthy with its high content of fiber and cholesterol-lowering properties. This recipe was a complete surprise to me—as was the patient who shared it. Originally from Louisiana, this patient appeared to be in her late seventies. I was amazed when I discovered she was actually ninety-nine years old! She walked without stooping, was clear in mind, looked youthful, and was dynamic in every way. I wanted to know what she ate to stay in such good shape, though I was a little skeptical of what recipes might come from Southern cuisine. She shared this pancake recipe, her favorite, which she eats almost every day and credits for her health and regularity.

SERVES 4

¾ cup buckwheat flour
½ cup gluten-free rolled oats
½ cup cornmeal
1 teaspoon baking powder
½ teaspoon baking soda
1 banana
2 tablespoons vinegar
2 cups almond milk
½ cup fresh blueberries
1 tablespoon grapeseed oil
   Maple syrup, for serving

1. In a medium bowl, whisk the flour, oats, cornmeal, baking powder, and baking soda together until combined. In a small bowl, mash the banana with the vinegar until smooth; whisk in the almond milk until well combined. Add the wet ingredients to the flour mixture and stir until just combined; do not overmix. Gently fold in the blueberries.

2. Heat the oil in a large nonstick skillet or griddle over medium heat. Ladle the batter, about ½ cup per pancake, onto the hot pan. Cook for 2 to 3 minutes, until bubbles appear on the surface and the underside is golden brown. Flip the pancakes and continue cooking until set and golden brown on the bottom, about 2 minutes more. Transfer the pancakes to a plate and cover to keep warm. Continue making pancakes until the batter is used up.

3. Serve the pancakes warm with maple syrup.

Buckwheat is not really a grain, but actually a fruit seed. A great source of fiber, manganese, and magnesium, and packed with B vitamins, buckwheat is also a good quality protein, containing the eight essential amino acids, including lysine, which is usually lacking in grains. With their rich contents of magnesium and fiber, whole grains like buckwheat can significantly lower your risk of cardiovascular disease, obesity, insulin resistance, and type 2 diabetes.

EGGLESS TOFU SCRAMBLE

BENEFITS: HEART + IMMUNITY + ANTI-INFLAMMATION + ANTI-AGING BEAUTY

This vegan breakfast is an excellent way to begin the day. With the tofu, you get a high-protein, low-fat meal packed with vital estrogen. These benefits make this a great choice for women, particularly those going through the change and beyond, as well as men with prostate issues. The celery lowers blood pressure and the antioxidant lycopene in the tomatoes helps defend against inflammation, cancer, and prostate issues. In addition, all these ingredients work together to help lower cholesterol and protect you from heart disease. Not bad for one meal!

SERVES 4

2   tablespoons water
3   stalks celery, chopped
12 button mushrooms, stemmed
    and sliced
1½ pounds firm tofu, cut into
    1-inch cubes and drained for 30
    minutes in a colander
2   medium tomatoes, diced
1   tablespoon avocado oil
    Salt and freshly ground black
    pepper
2   scallions, sliced, for garnish

Heat a large skillet with a lid over medium heat. When hot, add the water, celery, and mushrooms and cook, stirring, until the vegetables soften and begin to brown, 3 to 4 minutes. Add the tofu and tomatoes, stir well, and reduce the heat to medium-low. Cover the pan and cook for 5 minutes. Remove the lid, drizzle the oil evenly over the tofu, season with salt and pepper, and cook, stirring gently, until very hot, about 1 minute more. Remove from the heat, transfer to a serving plate, and sprinkle the scallions evenly over the top. Serve immediately.

Tofu was invented in second-century China from soybeans. Unlike other beans, soybeans are considered a source of complete protein, which include all the essential amino acids. In addition, soy has been researched for its potential ability to lower cardiovascular disease risk, reduce menopausal symptoms, aid in weight loss, treat arthritis, bolster brain function, and enhance exercise performance. Soy may decrease the risk of breast cancer and prostate cancer, as well as other types of cancers. That's several great reasons to start cooking with this versatile protein substitute!

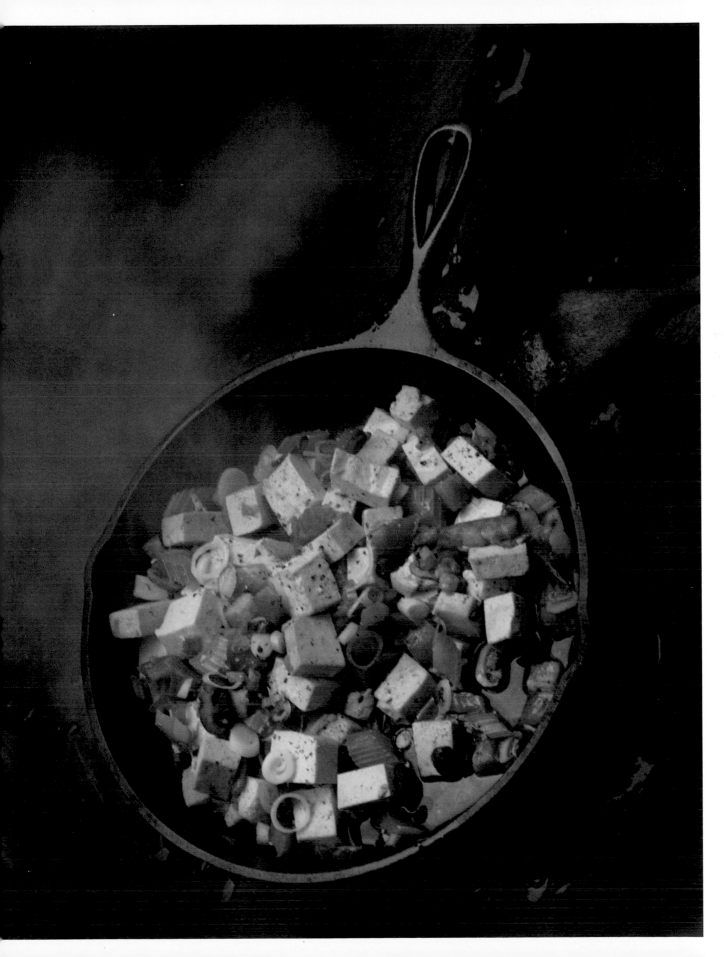

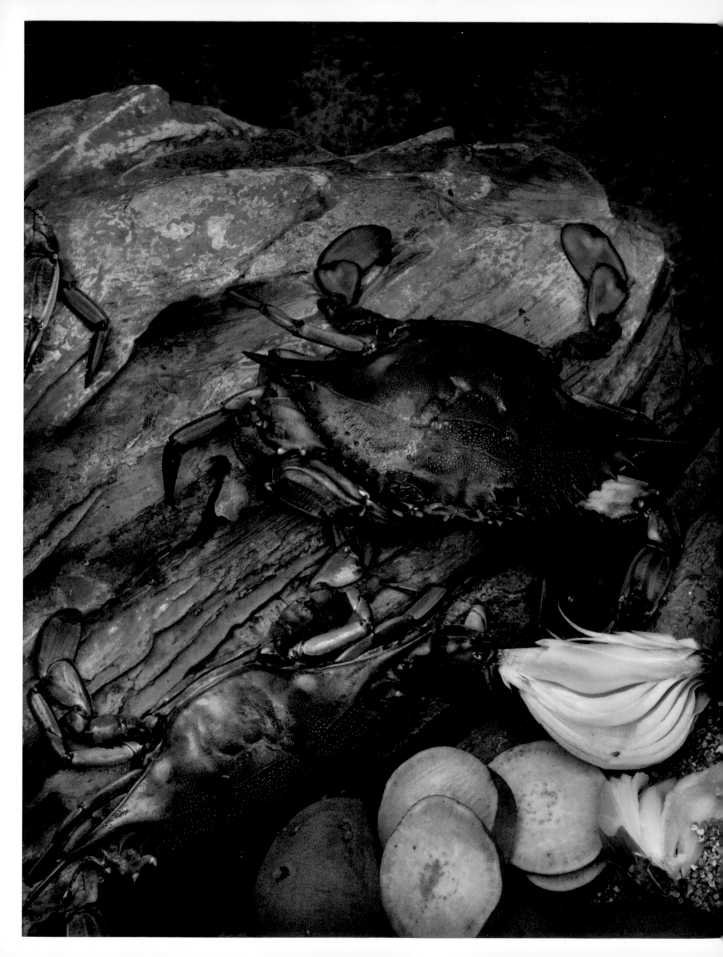

SWEET POTATO CRAB HASH

BENEFITS: ANTI-INFLAMMATION + METABOLISM + SEXUAL HEALTH

This is a wonderful variation on a favorite American breakfast food. During one of many trips to Maine, I stayed in a charming bed-and-breakfast that overlooked the rugged coast. The host, in her eighties, made this for breakfast. After one bite, I was smitten with the great taste, and I begged her for the recipe. After much persuasion, she finally relented—and now we can all be glad for it! Instead of the usual beef and potato that frequently make an appearance in hash browns, this version mixes crab, oats, and sweet potato with gourmet flair. Add in the egg whites and vegetables, and you've got an unforgettable breakfast that is super-healthy, to boot.

SERVES 4

2   large sweet potatoes, washed and scrubbed
1   cup steel-cut oats
1   cup frozen corn, thawed
½   sweet onion, finely chopped
2   scallions, finely chopped
1   teaspoon ground turmeric
½   teaspoon cayenne pepper
1   tablespoon almond oil
4   large egg whites
    Sea salt and freshly ground black pepper
12 ounces fresh crabmeat, picked over for shells and patted dry
3   sprigs fresh basil, for garnish

1. Preheat the oven to 350°F. Put the sweet potatoes on a baking sheet and roast until very tender, about 1 hour. Remove the sweet potatoes from oven but keep the oven on.

2. When cool enough to handle, peel the potatoes and mash the flesh with a fork in a mixing bowl. Add the oats, corn, onion, scallions, turmeric, cayenne, and almond oil and mix well until evenly combined. Add the egg whites, season with salt and pepper to taste, and mix well. Add the crabmeat and gently fold it into the mixture, being careful not to break the crab apart. Spread the hash mixture evenly in a small casserole dish and bake in the oven until very hot and completely cooked through, 40 to 45 minutes.

3. Garnish the hash with basil and serve directly from the casserole dish at the table.

Corn is an ancient crop, called *mahiz*, or "that which sustains us" by the North American indigenous people. Cooling in nature, corn is considered by traditional Chinese medicine to lower blood pressure, detoxify, and aid in the treatment of gallstones. Corn has heart-protective properties due to its fiber and significant folate (vitamin B_9) content. Folate also protects against colon cancer. Additionally, the thiamin (vitamin B_1) is thought to defend against Alzheimer's disease and age-related cognitive decline.

ASPARAGUS-ZUCCHINI BLOSSOM FRITTATA

BENEFITS: HEART + CLEANSING + DIGESTION + ANTI-AGING BEAUTY

A frittata, not to be confused with quiche, is an Italian-style omelet. Quiche has similar ingredients but usually packs in too much cheese and egg yolks to be very healthy. This version of a frittata is filled with vegetables, asparagus, sweet red peppers, and zucchini, but you can feel free to try your own variation with your favorite veggies.

SERVES 4

2 tablespoons avocado oil

8 ounces fresh or frozen asparagus, woody base discarded if using fresh, and cut into 1-inch long strips

1 small red bell pepper, cut into thin strips

2 medium zucchinis, halved lengthwise and cut into thin slices (about 1½ cups)

½ cup chopped sweet onion

2 cups egg whites, from about 12 eggs

½ cup soy milk

2 tablespoons tapioca flour

1 teaspoon fresh sage, finely chopped

1 teaspoon Heart Spice Blend, pg. 48 (cinnamon, fennel, clove, star anise, white pepper, parsley, ginger, cayenne, and turmeric)

½ teaspoon salt

½ teaspoon ground black pepper

8–10 zucchini blossoms

Cilantro sprigs, optional

1. Preheat oven to 350°F. Lightly coat a 2-quart rectangular baking dish with avocado oil; set aside.

2. Add 1 inch of water to a saucepan and bring to a boil. Add asparagus, bell pepper, zucchinis, and onion. Cover and simmer for 5 minutes; drain well. Spread asparagus-zucchini mixture evenly in baking dish.

3. In a mixing bowl, whisk together egg whites, soy milk, tapioca flour, sage, Heart Spice Blend, and salt and black pepper, until well mixed. Pour over vegetables in baking dish and place zucchini blossoms on top.

4. Bake, uncovered, for about 35 minutes, or until slightly puffed and top shakes slightly when dish is moved.

5. Let stand for 10 minutes before serving. If desired, garnish individual servings with cilantro sprigs.

With their high protein content, **eggs** will provide you with steady energy production for your whole day. Eggs are a source of all the B vitamins, including B_{12}, which is only found elsewhere in meat products. Additionally, lutein, a carotenoid that supports vision health, may be found in even higher amounts in eggs than in leafy green vegetables such as spinach. Although nutrition experts now suggest that one egg a day does not seem to adversely affect cholesterol levels, people on a low-cholesterol diet and those at risk for type 2 diabetes may need to reduce egg consumption. Keep a few hardboiled eggs in your refrigerator for an easy grab-and-go snack.

Chock full of vitamins A, C and K, folic acid, calcium, magnesium and potassium, **asparagus** is rich in the prebiotic inulin. (Prebiotics are non-digestible carbohydrates that promote a healthy living environment for your gut flora.) Approximately one cup of asparagus provides you with 3 grams of dietary fiber, which may lower your risk for heart disease and diabetes.

SOUPS

Soup is my favorite dish because it is one of the most effective ways to support your long-term health. Your immune system needs a lot of minerals to function properly and the typical Western diet does not always hit the mark. When you slowly simmer foods over low heat, you gently extract the energetic and therapeutic properties of the ingredients, preserving the nutritional value of the food. Even better, your body can very readily assimilate the nutrients in soups—more than any other type of prepared dish—because slow simmering has broken down the ingredients. It's important to know that boiling can destroy half of the vitamins found in vegetables, so cook soup over a low heat.

The soup recipes I have selected for this chapter are among the most powerful longevity recipes that I have come across in my many years of research, and their therapeutic benefits are as varied as the many regions they come from.

CLEANSING VEGETABLE BROTH

BENEFITS: HEART + CLEANSING

In our modern world, more heavy metals and pesticides are getting stored in our bodies than ever before, causing all sorts of disease. This powerful cleansing recipe not only cleans toxins from the body, but also replenishes minerals in the body with its rich content of potassium and magnesium. I discovered this recipe when I was looking for detoxification methods to reduce levels of mercury and other toxins in my own body. It originates from India and is attributed to an Ayurvedic doctor. As an interesting side note, this recipe turned up again in my research. In 10th century China, many people were falling ill from poisoning, caused by a mercury coating often used to beautify objects like spoons and utensils. It was such a problem that a school dedicated to mercury poisoning sprang up in China. As it happens, this recipe, slightly modified, was used to heal people suffering from poisoning. You know when two different health traditions have sworn by the same detoxifying recipe, you have time-tested benefits in store!

SERVES 8 TO 10

1   bunch Swiss chard, chopped
1   bunch kale, chopped
1   bunch mustard greens, chopped
½   head white cabbage, chopped
1   bunch dandelion greens, chopped
1   cup Brussels sprouts, chopped
1   large daikon radish, diced
1   bunch watercress, chopped
4   ounces kombu or wakame seaweed
6   dried shiitake mushrooms
2   cloves garlic, crushed
2   leeks, sliced
1   fennel bulb, chopped
1   4-inch piece fresh ginger, peeled and chopped
1   teaspoon ground star anise
1   teaspoon ground turmeric
1   bunch fresh parsley, chopped
1   bunch fresh cilantro, chopped
    Chicken stock, as needed, optional
    Red chili flakes, optional

1. Put all of the ingredients into a large stockpot and fill it with enough water to cover vegetables but at least 2 inches below the rim of pot. Set the pot over medium-high heat and bring to a boil; reduce the heat to medium-low and simmer for 1 hour.

2. Using a mesh strainer, remove the vegetables and set aside. Continue cooking the broth for an additional 15 minutes to strengthen the flavor and reduce slightly.

3. Let the broth cool completely in the pot before transferring to glass jars. Store in the refrigerator for up to 1 week, or freeze in airtight plastic containers for up to 1 month.

4. Reheat before serving.

5. For cleansing and detoxification, consume 3 cups a day.

NOTE: If you want to use the cooked vegetables, working in batches, puree them in a food processor or blender with just enough chicken stock to liquefy them and then transfer the puree to a saucepan. Heat over medium-low heat until warmed; ladle into bowls and garnish with chili flakes. Serve immediately.

Considered a liver tonic by practitioners of traditional Chinese medicine, **dandelion** is said to enhance the flow of bile in your body, improving the function of your liver, and remedying liver conditions such as gallstones and jaundice. These leafy greens are also full of vitamin C, higher in beta-carotene than carrots, and richer in iron and calcium content than spinach.

SQUASH PEANUT SOUP

BENEFITS: ANTI-INFLAMMATION + BRAIN & VISION + GOOD MOOD

My mother has been making this sweet, creamy squash and peanut combination for as long as I can remember, often at my request. The recipe was passed down in her family. Her grandparents, who ate this soup frequently, lived well into their nineties. The peanuts are high in protein and contain an incredible amount of nutrients. In fact, during my studies of centenarian diets, peanuts were one of the top ten longevity foods, particularly when cooked, as they become more digestible than when raw. The squash is filled with fiber, vitamin A, and B complex. This is a wonderful soup for all seasons, but its heartiness makes it especially satisfying in the winter.

SERVES 4

1 cup dried, shelled peanuts, soaked overnight in 2 cups filtered water

4 cups filtered water

1 small daikon radish, diced into bite-size cubes

½ small kabocha squash (Japanese pumpkin), diced into bite-size cubes

1 medium carrot, diced into bite-size cubes

2 teaspoons Anti-Inflammatory Spice Blend, pg. 48 (basil, black pepper, cinnamon, chili powder, cloves, curry, fennel, marjoram, nutmeg, oregano, rosemary, sage, tarragon)

2 tablespoons cilantro, chopped

1. Pour the peanuts and soaking water into a saucepan, add the 4 cups of additional water, and bring to a boil over medium-high heat. Reduce the heat to medium-low, cover, and simmer the peanuts for 1 hour.

2. Add the radish and squash pieces, cover, and simmer for 30 minutes, or until tender. Add the carrots, cover, and cook an additional 15 minutes. Remove the soup from the heat, stir in the Anti-Inflammatory Spice Blend and the cilantro. Serve immediately.

Peanuts are not actually nuts at all, but a member of the legume "bean" family Fabaceae, which includes peas and lentils. Even so, peanuts contain more protein than any true nut. In traditional Chinese medicine, peanuts are used to improve appetite, regulate blood flow, alleviate insomnia, and treat edema. Peanuts protect heart health with their monounsaturated fats, vitamin E, folate, magnesium, and manganese. As a good source of niacin, peanuts contribute to brain health and blood flow, giving protection against Alzheimer's disease and age-related cognitive decline.

VEGETARIAN HOT AND SOUR SOUP

BENEFITS: HEART + IMMUNITY + ANTI-INFLAMMATION

Hot and sour soup is famous in Chinese cuisine. This is a vegan version of the classic, similar to the one my mother used to make for my father, who has been vegetarian for many years. This amazing array of ingredients helps promote circulation, purify the blood, and defend against cancer. Do not miss out on the benefits by skimping on the lily blossom and wood ear mushroom— it just wouldn't be the same healing soup without them. You can easily find these items in an Asian market or online. Look at it as an adventure in healing and an investment in your good health!

SERVES 6

½ handful kombu seaweed

½ cup dried lily blossoms

½ cup dried wood ear mushrooms

5 dried shiitake mushrooms

6 cups filtered water

⅓ pound firm tofu, cut into matchsticks

½ cup julienned carrots

½ cup julienned jicama

2 large eggs, beaten

1 tablespoon rice vinegar

½ teaspoon freshly ground black pepper

2 teaspoons arrowroot powder

2 tablespoons water

1 teaspoon toasted sesame oil

1 tablespoon chopped cilantro leaves, for garnish

1. Rinse the seaweed, lily blossoms, and wood ear and shiitake mushrooms under cold running water and transfer them to a large bowl. Fill the bowl with fresh water and soak the ingredients for 2 hours.

2. Drain the water and slice the seaweed, lily blossoms and mushrooms into thin strips, discarding the stems. Transfer them to a large saucepan and add the 6 cups of water. Bring to a boil over medium-high heat, then reduce the heat to medium-low and simmer for 30 minutes, or until tender.

3. Increase the heat to medium and add the tofu, carrots, and jicama, and cook for 2 minutes. While stirring constantly, drizzle in the eggs and cook for 2 more minutes; add the vinegar and black pepper. In a small bowl, stir the arrowroot powder and water together until dissolved; gently stir it into the soup. Continue cooking, stirring gently, until the soup returns to a simmer and thickens.

4. Remove the soup from the heat, drizzle the sesame oil over the top and garnish with the cilantro. Serve hot.

The brown, ear-shaped **wood ear mushroom** frequently appears in hot and sour soup recipes. They are popular in Chinese cooking for their mild taste and health benefits, which include incredible anti-cancer, anti-inflammatory, and antioxidant properties. In herbalism, these mushrooms have traditionally been used to promote blood circulation and help treat diabetes and cancer. Wood ear mushrooms, also called "mo-er," can be found in dried form, often pre-sliced, online and in Asian markets. *Consult your physician before trying a new food, especially if you are pregnant or taking medication.*

SEAWEED MISO SOUP

BENEFITS: ANTI-INFLAMMATION + DIGESTION + ANTI-AGING BEAUTY

An eighty-two-year-old patient of mine from Okinawa shared this Japanese recipe with me. She ate this soup nearly every morning with brown rice for breakfast, which may sound like an odd choice if you are used to cereal, eggs, or bacon—but look at the incredible nutritious profile of this soup! The nori seaweed per gram contains more calcium than cheese, more iron than beef, and more protein than eggs. Miso is high in protein and fiber, and boasts a wide array of protective antioxidants. This rich broth is very easy to digest, great for people with digestion that takes a little time to wake up in the morning. Paired with brown rice, you will be totally satisfied. Be adventurous and try a Japanese breakfast! After all, people in Okinawa are some of the longest living people in the world, due in large part to their healthy diet.

SERVES 4

4	cups filtered water
½	pound firm tofu, cut into bite-sized cubes
¼	cup frozen peas, thawed
1	small tomato, chopped
2 to 3	tablespoons low-sodium miso, dissolved in 2 tablespoons water
1	sheet nori seaweed, torn into small pieces
1	tablespoon minced scallions
1	teaspoon toasted sesame oil

Bring the 4 cups of water to a boil in a deep saucepan over medium-high heat. Add the tofu and cook for 2 minutes; stir in the peas, tomatoes, and dissolved miso paste and cook for 1 minute. Turn off the heat, add the seaweed and scallions, and stir well. Drizzle the sesame oil over the soup and serve immediately.

Best known as the outer wrap of sushi rolls, **nori** is a great food for skin health. Just one sheet of nori has the same amount of omega-3s as two whole avocados. Omega-3s boost cardiovascular health and also create a natural oil barrier on your skin, helping to reduce acne and dry skin. Nori also helps reduce the body's production of inflammatory compounds that affect how healthy the skin looks and feels. Find nori in Asian grocery stores and health-food stores.

IMMUNITY-BOOSTING BORSCHT WITH PORCINI MUSHROOMS

BENEFITS: IMMUNITY + ANTI-INFLAMMATION + BRAIN & VISION

I had a Polish patient who passed away at age 100, and both of her parents lived to 100. This was a dish they ate throughout the year, especially around holidays. They traditionally celebrated Christmas dinner with a clear broth borscht soup. I have modified the recipe slightly by including the whole mushroom instead of just the broth because porcini mushrooms are such a wonderful healing food, both tasty and good for your immune system. Beets contain powerful anti-inflammatory and antioxidant properties, thanks to betalains, the pigment that gives them their deep red hue. With its festive color and immune-boosting qualities, you will want to celebrate your good health!

SERVES 4

2	medium-size bunches of red beets with leaves, rinsed well
2	medium onions
3	medium carrots
3	stalks celery
2 to 3	garlic cloves
8	ounces dried porcini mushrooms
1	(15-ounce) can tomato sauce
1	tablespoon powdered chicken bouillon
	Salt and freshly ground pepper

1. Peel the beets and push them through a juicer, along with the leaves, onions, carrots, celery, and garlic; reserve the juice. Remove the pulp from the juicer, transfer it to a large skillet, and add just enough water to cover. Bring the pulp to a simmer over medium heat and cook for 20 minutes. Pour the mixture through a fine mesh strainer set over a bowl and discard the pulp. Combine the cooked liquid with the reserved fresh juice and set aside.

2. Meanwhile, put the mushrooms into another large skillet and add just enough water to cover. Bring to a boil over medium heat and cook until tender, about 30 minutes. Using a slotted spoon, transfer the mushrooms to a cutting board and let stand until cool enough to handle. Discard the mushroom cooking liquid.

3. Finely chop the mushrooms and return them to the skillet. Add the liquid beet mixture, tomato sauce, and bouillon and bring the mixture to a boil over medium-high heat. Reduce the heat to medium-low and simmer the soup for 15 minutes, stirring occasionally; season with salt and pepper to taste. Ladle the soup into bowls and serve.

Beets are an all-in-one superfood! The colorful beetroots contain powerful nutrients that help protect against heart disease, birth defects, and cancer, especially colon cancer. This ruby root may also protect liver cells from harmful chemicals with an antioxidant compound called betacyanin. Beet greens are nutrient-rich in beta-carotene and lutein, helpful for vision health. The greens are also high in potassium and contain high levels of folic acid, which can help ward off certain birth defects and lung cancer.

IMMUNITY SOUP

BENEFITS: IMMUNITY + ANTI-INFLAMMATION + METABOLISM + CLEANSING + DIGESTION + GOOD MOOD

This recipe came from a patient whose mother had stage IV lung cancer and survived it, all because of this soup. They received this recipe from a very famous cancer doctor in China. She was in her seventies when diagnosed, but after drinking this soup, remarkably went into remission and lived into her late eighties. Just take a look at these powerful ingredients! Mushrooms are known to increase natural killer cell activity, especially shiitake, which, although it doesn't outright heal cancer, can give additional support. Mung beans are a major detoxifier, while jujube dates are good for building blood. This soup can also solve the problem of appetite loss that often accompanies cancer treatment, with its tasty healing herbs that help stimulate appetite, settle the stomach, and boost energy.

SERVES 4

½ cup dried soybeans
½ cup lentils
½ cup dried mung beans
10 pieces dried shiitake mushrooms
10 dried red jujube dates
2 onions, chopped
1 head garlic, cloves separated and peeled
2 leeks, trimmed and chopped
2 cups fresh dandelion greens
6 to 8 slices fresh ginger, peeled
5 scallions, chopped
1 teaspoon ground turmeric
1 teaspoon freshly ground black pepper
1 teaspoon cinnamon
1 teaspoon ground cardamom
1 teaspoon ground cloves
1 bunch parsley, chopped
1 tablespoon chopped fresh cilantro
1 teaspoon chopped fresh rosemary
1 teaspoon chopped fresh basil
1 teaspoon chopped fresh chives
   Cooked brown rice, for serving

1. Put all of the ingredients except the rice into a large stockpot. Fill the pot with water to within an inch of the top and bring it to a boil over medium-high heat. Reduce the heat to medium-low and simmer uncovered, stirring occasionally, until the dried beans are soft, at least 2 hours and up to 3 hours.

2. Serve the soup with brown rice. Let the soup cool to room temperature before storing in the refrigerator in airtight containers for up to 3 days. Reheat when ready to eat.

In traditional Chinese medicine **jujube dates** are often prescribed to cancer patients, to help them manage the anemia that can come from chemotherapy. Red jujube dates are traditionally used as a medicinal aid to people suffering from chronic illness or fatigue and to women after giving birth. They help rebuild blood by stimulating kidney and bone marrow functions, and they will raise energy levels, calm the mind, and balance hormones. Find them in Asian markets, some health-food stores, and online.

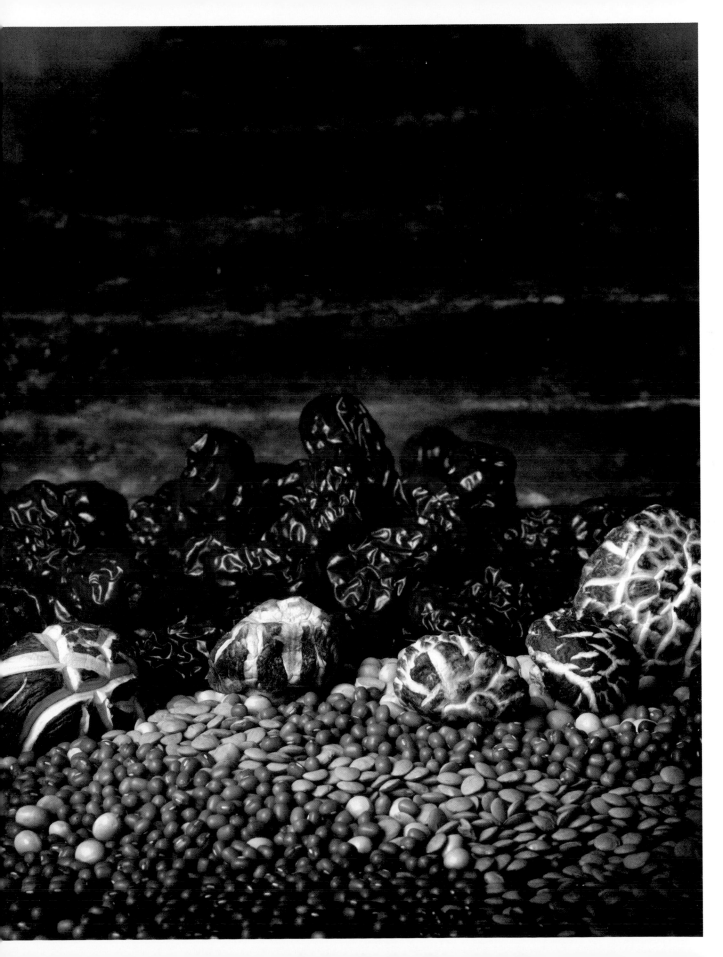

IMMUNITY-BOOSTING CREAM OF MUSHROOM AND CAULIFLOWER SOUP

BENEFITS: IMMUNITY + BRAIN & VISION

For mushroom lovers, there's nothing like a hearty, creamy cup of mushroom soup seasoned with herbs. This recipe combines the wonderfully intense flavors of shiitake and portobello mushrooms with cilantro, oregano, garlic, and onion, a collection of ingredients that work synergistically to boost your immunity to colds and flu and also act like natural antibiotics to help you fight infection. Best of all, the cream base for the soup is dairy-free and uses the natural, creamy texture of cauliflower, a cruciferous vegetable that helps prevent cancer.

SERVES 4

2 tablespoons olive oil
1 medium onion, chopped
2 cloves garlic, crushed
1 small head cauliflower, cut into bite-size pieces
5 cups chicken stock
½ cup fresh shiitake mushrooms, coarsely chopped
½ cup portobello mushrooms, coarsely chopped
½ cup white button mushrooms, coarsely chopped
½ cup white wine
½ cup chopped fresh cilantro
   Salt and freshly ground pepper
   Fresh oregano sprigs, for garnish

1. Heat the oil in a large saucepan over medium heat. Stir in the onion, garlic, and cauliflower; reduce heat to low, cover, and cook until the onion and cauliflower are softened, 8 to 10 minutes. Add the stock, mushrooms, wine, and three-quarters of the cilantro. Bring the soup to a boil and cook over medium heat until the mushrooms are softened, about 15 minutes. Remove from the heat and let cool.

2. Working in batches, puree the soup in a food processor or blender until smooth. Return the soup to a clean saucepan and bring it to a simmer over medium heat; season with salt and pepper to taste.

3. To serve, ladle the warm soup into serving bowls and sprinkle the remaining cilantro over the top. Garnish with oregano sprigs, if desired.

Cauliflower is a great alternative to dairy products, especially when you want to use a cream base for soups and sauces. With its mild taste, it blends easily into other dishes. Like other cruciferous vegetables, cauliflower is a rich source of phytonutrients that help cleanse the body of cancer-causing substances and provide significant cardiovascular benefits. In folklore, cauliflower is thought to be beneficial for mental function, owing to its similar appearance to the brain. Indeed, it is a good source of the B vitamin choline, an essential nutrient for memory and brain health. With so many benefits to gain, why would you ever make a dairy-based cream again?

CREAMY SWEET POTATO SOUP

BENEFITS: HEART + IMMUNITY + METABOLISM + BRAIN & VISION

The sweet potato, which stars in this centenarian recipe from China, is on the top-ten list of longevity foods. In my own extensive research, I found that sweet potatoes showed up with great frequency in the diets of Chinese centenarians. This orange root vegetable is rich in vitamin A, as well as plant sterols, which have cholesterol-lowering properties. Sweet potatoes also offer support to people with insulin resistance or diabetes. So if I were you, I would put them on your top-ten list, too!

SERVES 4

1   small head cauliflower, chopped into small chunks
1   tablespoon grapeseed oil
1   small white onion, chopped
2   pounds sweet potatoes, peeled and cut into bite-size cubes
2   firm pears, peeled, cored, and cut into bite-size cubes
4   cups vegetable stock
1   teaspoon Heart Spice Blend, pg. 48 (cinnamon, fennel, clove, star anise, white pepper, parsley, ginger, cayenne, and turmeric)
    Salt and freshly ground pepper
    Fresh mint leaves, for garnish

1. Put the cauliflower and 2 cups of water into a saucepan, bring to a boil, and cook until the cauliflower is very soft, about 10 minutes. Drain and transfer the cauliflower into a blender or food processor and puree until creamy. Set aside in a bowl.

2. Heat the grapeseed oil in a saucepan over medium heat. Add the onions and cook for 2 minutes, until softened. Add the sweet potatoes and pears, stir well, and cook for an additional 2 minutes. Add the stock to the pan and bring the soup to a boil. Reduce the heat to medium-low and simmer for 20 minutes, or until the sweet potato is soft. Remove from the heat and let cool.

3. Working in batches, puree the soup in a blender or food processor until smooth. Return the soup to the pan, stir in the cauliflower cream, and reheat gently over medium-low heat; do not boil. Add the Heart Spice Blend 1 minute before turning off the heat. Season with salt and pepper, to taste; garnish with mint and serve.

The tasty **sweet potato**, which gets its color from its carotenoid antioxidant compounds, helps defend against free radicals, improving eyesight and bolstering the immune system. Sweet potatoes contain higher amounts of beta-carotene and vitamin C than carrots, more protein than rice, and more fiber than oat bran. Sweet potatoes help balance the glycemic index in the body, which controls how the body responds to the food you eat. When someone has an insulin resistance condition, their body responds to everything they eat by creating more insulin than needed, increasing risk for type 2 diabetes, rapid aging, cancer, and other diseases. Luckily, eating sweet potatoes can help slow this process down. Start eating more of this orange powerhouse to get all the sweet benefits!

SPRING SOUP

BENEFITS: ANTI-INFLAMMATION + METABOLISM + CLEANSING

As the name would suggest, this soup is perfect to eat in the spring, just when your body is most naturally poised for cleansing. This soup, traditionally eaten in China as a springtime ritual, has natural detoxifying properties, mainly deriving from the watercress. Watercress has natural diuretic properties that help you release excess fluids, which often contain toxins and waste products. Of course, feel free to eat this soup for cleansing any time of year!

SERVES 2

1   turnip, cut into thin 1-inch strips
2   stalks celery, cut into thin 1-inch strips
1   carrot, cut into thin 1-inch strips
1   scallion, cut into thin 1-inch strips
½   pound watercress
3   quarter-size slices of fresh ginger, peeled and cut crosswise into very thin strips
1   cooked chicken breast or ¼ pound extra-firm tofu, cut into 1-inch cubes
2   cups chicken or vegetable stock
2   cups water
    Salt

1. Combine all of the ingredients, except the salt, in a large pot and bring to a boil over medium-high heat. Reduce the heat to low, and simmer, covered, for 40 minutes, or until the vegetables are soft.

2. Taste and season with salt, if desired. Serve the soup immediately. It is best served when freshly made—the therapeutic value decreases the longer the soup sits.

The use of **watercress** can be traced back over three millennia to the Persians, Greeks, and Romans and was used for everything from increasing strength to remedying stomach ailments. For weight loss, it is also a natural diuretic that helps alleviate a bloated sensation and excess water retention. Watercress has been linked to a reduction of DNA damage caused by free radicals and a reduction in blood triglycerides. As a member of the cabbage family, watercress boasts an incredible nutrient profile that includes vitamins A, B_6, C, E, and K as well as calcium, iron, magnesium, zinc, and the potent flavonoid, quercetin, which serves as a natural anti-inflammatory. Don't underestimate these small, leafy greens the next time you hit the grocery store!

SUMMER VEGETABLE SOUP

BENEFITS: HEART + IMMUNITY

This traditional Chinese recipe is specially designed to get you through the summer months in good health. The ingredients in this soup are summer seasonal veggies—and they are cooling in nature, in spite of the fact that you are eating them in warm soup. Collectively, the vitamin- and fiber-rich ingredients in this soup help to actually cool your system. This soup helps you easily hit the healthy target of seven servings of vegetables a day, helping lower your risk for heart disease, stroke, and cancer.

SERVES 4

1   onion, chopped
2   carrots, chopped
1   clove garlic, finely chopped
1   zucchini, cut into ¼-inch dice
2   tomatoes, chopped
1   handful green beans, trimmed
    and cut into ¼-inch slices
1   cup fresh corn kernels
1   cup tomato sauce
1   teaspoon Cleansing Spice Blend,
    pg. 48 (turmeric, ground ginger,
    dried parsley, dried rosemary,
    cayenne pepper, fenugreek, and
    fennel seed)
    Tamari
¼   cup finely chopped fresh cilantro,
    for garnish
¼   cup finely chopped fresh chives,
    for garnish

1. Bring 2 quarts of water to a boil in a stockpot over medium-high heat. Add the onion, carrots, garlic, zucchini, tomatoes, green beans, and corn. Reduce the heat to low and simmer, covered, for about 30 minutes, or until the vegetables are tender.

2. Stir in the tomato sauce and cook until warmed through. Add the Cleansing Spice Blend 1 minute before turning off the heat. Season the soup with herb salt and tamari to taste. Ladle into serving bowls and garnish the soup with cilantro and chives.

Traditional Chinese medicine usually does not recommend **raw food**, as it is thought to put out the digestive fire and cause stomach issues. This is particularly true in the summer, when the hot weather heats your body up, leaving you more at risk of inflammation and infection. Also, during hot weather, parasites and microorganisms proliferate, making it much easier for us to get sick from affected produce and meat—unless we sterilize by cooking. Cooking also makes the nutrients in food easier to assimilate for your body. So, though it may seem counterintuitive in the hotter months, I heartily recommend you support your health with a delicious soup!

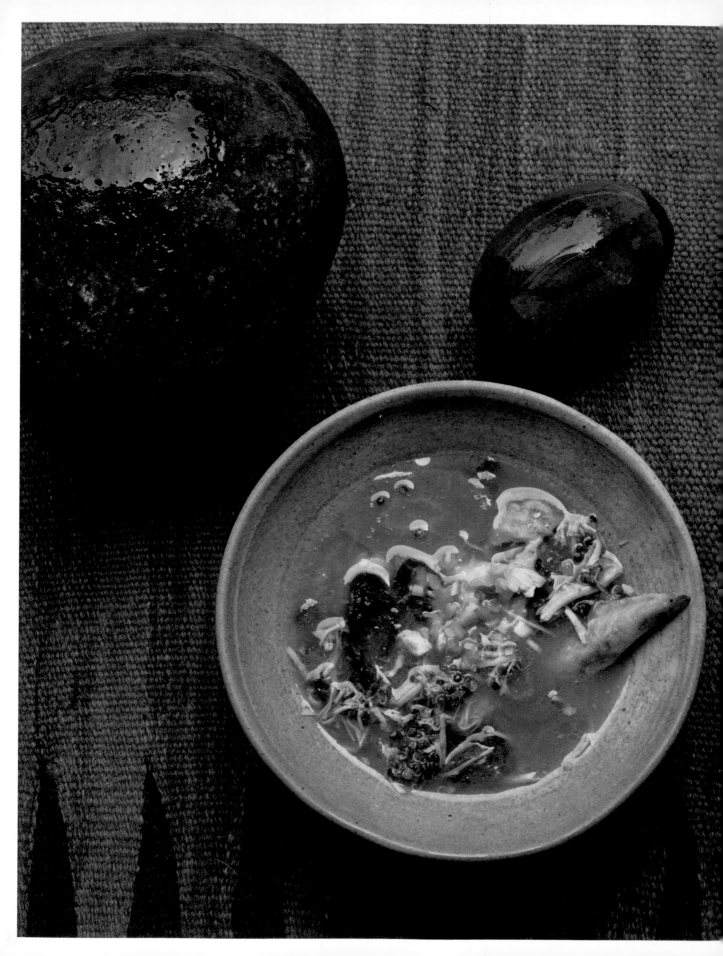

CHICKEN LEEK SOUP WITH DRIED PLUMS AND QUINOA

BENEFITS: HEART + METABOLISM + DIGESTION

This delicious dish combines the natural sweetness of dried plums with the pungent leek for a wonderful fusion of unique flavors and healthy benefits. A French-Canadian patient of mine from Montreal shared this recipe, which had been passed down in her family, a dish they often ate for Canadian Thanksgiving instead of turkey. My patient claimed it was her grandmother's favorite, who lived to be 102. Combining the dried plums with the chicken helps break down the proteins, making this dish easier to digest. The plum itself has numerous benefits, including that it is high in vitamins, good for digestion, and helps keep the chicken moist. Quinoa is very high in protein and fiber, plus it cooks fast, tastes delicious, and is a very nice complement to the chicken.

SERVES 8

1   (4-pound) whole chicken
10 cups low-sodium chicken stock
1   pound leeks, trimmed and thinly sliced
3   stalks lemongrass, smashed
2   stalks celery, coarsely chopped
1   large carrot, sliced
½   cup quinoa
1   teaspoon salt
1   teaspoon freshly ground black pepper
1   pound pitted California dried plums (prunes), sliced
1   scallion, chopped, for garnish

1. Rinse the chicken and put it in a large stockpot along with the stock, leeks, lemongrass, celery, and carrot. Bring to a boil over medium-high heat; reduce the heat and simmer for 30 minutes. Skim off any fat that rises to the surface.

2. Carefully remove the chicken and transfer it to a cutting board. When cool enough to handle, remove the meat from the bones (discard carcass and skin).

3. Rinse the quinoa in a strainer under cold running water; drain and add it to the stockpot. Bring the soup to a boil; reduce the heat and simmer until the quinoa is soft and fluffy, about 15 minutes, skimming off any fat that rises to the surface. Remove and discard the lemongrass. Stir in the salt and pepper.

4. Cut the chicken breast into thin strips and add it to the stockpot, along with the dried plums (reserve remaining chicken for another use). Simmer the soup for 5 more minutes.

5. To serve, ladle the hot soup into bowls and garnish with scallions

Packed with vitamin C and essential minerals like potassium and magnesium, **dried plums**—better known as prunes to some—contain a perfectly balanced proportion of soluble and insoluble fibers, ensuring bowel regularity, protecting against high cholesterol and heart disease, and preventing insulin resistance, making them an effective aid for weight management and diabetes care. Dried plums are very helpful for anemic people who may be experiencing the constipation that comes from taking iron supplements. A few dried plums a day help prevent constipation, a trait for which the dried plum has always been famous!

CHINESE WILD YAM AND PUMPKIN PUREE WITH GINGER

BENEFITS: ANTI-INFLAMMATION + METABOLISM + DIGESTION + SEXUAL HEALTH

This Chinese recipe features potent healing food that will endow you with strong vitality that can help prevent premature aging. Chinese wild yam—not to be confused with the regular yam you see in the produce section—increases stamina and ginger promotes digestion. Combined with pumpkin, this is a great dish for diabetes, because these ingredients work together to balance insulin and blood sugar levels, and also maintain steady energy.

SERVES 4

½   pound dried Chinese wild yam, soaked in hot water for 1 hour (if using fresh, 1 pound, unsoaked)

2   pounds pumpkin (kabocha squash or Japanese pumpkin) peeled, seeded, and cut into wedges

4   ounces elephant garlic cloves, peeled

3   tablespoons olive oil

1   teaspoon salt, plus more as needed

1   tablespoon granulated sugar

1   sweet onion, chopped

1   tablespoon grated fresh ginger

2   tablespoons miso paste, dissolved in 5 cups hot water
    Salt and freshly ground black pepper

1. Preheat the oven to 375°F. Brush the wild yam, pumpkin and garlic with 2 tablespoons of the olive oil and sprinkle with salt and sugar. Roast on a baking sheet for 30 minutes, or until soft. Remove the vegetables from the oven and set aside.

2. Heat the remaining oil in a skillet over medium heat, add the onion, and cook until softened, about 5 minutes. Remove from the heat.

3. Working in batches in a food processor, puree the roasted yam, pumpkin, and garlic with the onion, ginger, and enough miso broth to liquefy. Transfer the mixture, as you puree it, into a saucepan, along with any miso broth that is left. Stir and season the soup with salt and pepper, to taste. Reheat the soup gently over medium-low heat; do not boil. Serve in warmed bowls.

Chinese wild yam, also known as radix dioscorea, is not the same as your usual yam. It is considered a healing herb in traditional Chinese medicine, usually eaten for energy, vitality, improved hormonal function, and for the benefit of the digestive system, spleen, and pancreas. Wild yam is rich in DHEA, the precursor hormone to estrogen, progesterone, and testosterone; low levels of DHEA are associated with muscle weakness, joint pain, and depression. It is also useful to stabilize blood sugar and relieve inflammation. You can find it fresh in select Asian markets or in dried form online.

CHICKEN MANGO AND BUTTERNUT SQUASH SOUP

BENEFITS: HEART + IMMUNITY + ANTI-INFLAMMATION + BRAIN & VISION + SEXUAL HEALTH

A friend from Thailand shared this delicious soup recipe with me. Thai cuisine often features a wide array of herbs and spices, all of which help promote longevity due to their volatile oil content. These spices help dilate blood vessels, which is supportive for brain health, immunity, hormonal function, and high blood pressure. The mango not only gives this soup its wonderful flavor, but also contains enzymes that help break proteins in chicken, making it easier to digest the nutrients in the soup. According to my friend, this recipe was a favorite of his grandparents, who were in their late nineties at the time he shared the recipe.

SERVES 4

2   teaspoons toasted sesame oil
1   medium onion, sliced
1   small butternut squash, peeled, seeded, and diced
1   mango, peeled, pitted, and diced
2   teaspoons grated fresh ginger
1   clove garlic, finely chopped
1   red chili pepper, finely chopped
4   cups chicken stock
2   tablespoons freshly squeezed lime juice
1   pound boneless, skinless chicken breast, sliced into thin strips
1   tablespoon chopped fresh cilantro, for garnish

1. Heat the oil in a deep saucepan over medium-high heat; add the onion and cook for 5 minutes, or until golden. Stir in the squash and cook for another 5 minutes. Add the mango, ginger, garlic, and chili, and stir. Pour in the stock and lime juice and bring to a boil. Reduce the heat to medium and simmer for 20 minutes.

2. Add the chicken to the simmering broth and cook for 5 minutes, until just cooked through. Garnish with cilantro and serve the soup hot.

A close cousin to the pumpkin, **butternut squash** has a sweet flavor and is rich in vitamins A, B, and C. Butternut squash has very high content of beta-carotene, which has powerful antioxidant and anti-inflammatory properties that help combat cancer, heart disease, and cataracts. Beta-carotene also prevents the oxidation of cholesterol in the vessels; in other words, no plaque develops that can cause restricted blood flow and lead to heart disease. Serve up all the heart-health benefits that come with this beautiful squash!

SAFFRON GINGER FISH SOUP

BENEFITS: HEART + ANTI-INFLAMMATION + DIGESTION

I first tried this soup in Singapore, at a special dinner hosted by a woman whose family had emigrated from Southeast Asia. It was so soothing to my stomach because of the ginger. The saffron creates a wonderful, bold, yellow-colored broth, which I mistook for curry at first glance. It turns out there's more than one way to create a colorful broth! Saffron also has medicinal properties, one of which is that it promotes circulation. The hostess told me that it was her father's favorite soup and that she believed this specific soup had benefited his heart health. The saffron and ginger activate blood circulation, making this the perfect food for supporting someone with a heart condition.

SERVES 4

3 cups chicken stock

2 cups white wine

1 3-inch piece galangal root or fresh ginger, sliced

1 teaspoon saffron threads

2 teaspoons almond oil

1 onion, chopped

1 carrot, chopped

1 stalk celery, chopped

2 pounds firm boneless, skinless, white fish fillets, such as cod or bass, cut into cubes

2 tablespoons arrowroot powder

2 tablespoons water

Salt and freshly ground black pepper

Parsley sprigs, for garnish

1. Put the stock, wine, galangal, and saffron threads into a large saucepan and bring to a boil over medium-high heat. Reduce the heat to medium-low and simmer for 20 minutes.

2. Meanwhile, heat the oil in a skillet over medium heat and add the onion, carrot, and celery; cook until softened, 3 to 4 minutes. Remove from the heat.

3. Remove the galangal from the broth and discard. Add the fish and cooked vegetables to the simmering broth and cook for 2 minutes. In a small bowl, stir the arrowroot together with 2 tablespoons of water until dissolved; slowly stir the mixture into the soup and add salt and pepper to taste. Simmer for 2 to 3 minutes, until fish is cooked through and broth is thickened.

4. Garnish with the parsley and serve the hot soup immediately.

Famous in the West for relieving nausea, **ginger** has been used by Chinese doctors since ancient times to fire up vitality and cure body aches, such as arthritis, headaches, menstrual cramps, and muscle soreness. Ginger—also known as "galangal" or "galanga"—has been found to contain geraniol, which may be a potent cancer fighter. It also possesses anti-inflammatory properties that help alleviate pain and prevent blood clots. People on blood thinners and other medications should take extra precaution with this natural blood-thinner.

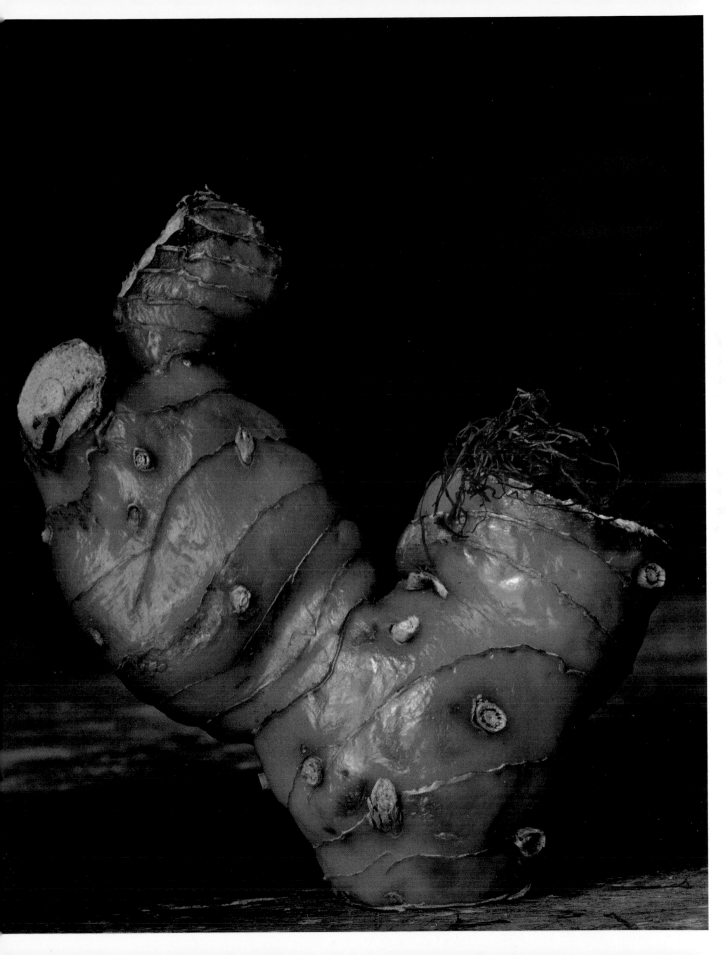

SALADS

The U.S. has a love affair with salads, and it's not hard to see why when they combine such tasty, nutritious produce with such refreshing, crisp textures. You will notice that many of these salads feature fruits and vegetables that grow in warm climates or are harvested in the summer: cucumbers, watermelon, mint. Mother Nature has the perfect plan for providing food that your body needs for each season, and most of these salad recipes include cooling ingredients that are perfect to eat during hot, steamy days. I live in Los Angeles, which is no stranger to salad, but on the East Coast, there is a particular zest for salads in the summer, and you will see that many of the recipes in this section come from that region.

The salads I selected for this section were ones that I very much enjoyed eating, but I do want to mention that in traditional Chinese medicine, eating raw or chilled food is usually discouraged, as it is said to dampen your digestive function, which is discussed in more detail on page 49. One other thing to consider about raw food is that it may potentially harbor microorganisms that could make you sick, so be sure to clean your produce well and follow proper prep methods, as outlined on page 43. With those caveats in mind, savor the flavor of nature's bounty in these salad recipes!

ORANGE FRUIT SALAD WITH MAPLE-GLAZED GINGER PECANS

BENEFITS: HEART + IMMUNITY + BRAIN & VISION

When I was traveling in Vermont, I came across this salad at a small country inn that the whole family lived in. I loved it so much that I asked for the recipe. The family brought out their grandparents, who were in their nineties. Apparently this high-fiber salad had been serving the family healthy and happy benefits for a long time! And it makes sense. The citrus fruits are full of vitamin C and bioflavonoids. The apples contain pectin, which lowers cholesterol and gives your intestines a nice sweep. Pecans contain lots of essential fatty acids that benefit brain and heart health. Throw in the Vermont maple syrup, and you have a sweet, light fruit salad that is perfect for a hot summer day, satisfying but not too heavy.

SERVES 4

3 to 4 navel oranges
1   green apple, washed, cored, and diced
1   red apple, washed, cored, and diced
½   cup freshly squeezed orange juice
1   cup plain soy or coconut yogurt
2   tablespoons honey
½   cup pecan halves
¼   cup maple syrup
2   tablespoons chopped fresh ginger

1. Peel 3 of the oranges and reserve 1 whole peel for garnish. Separate the sections and cut out any seeds and discard them. Cut the oranges into small chunks and put them in a strainer set over a pitcher or bowl to catch the juice while you prepare the rest of the fruit.

2. Put the diced apples and orange pieces into a bowl. Pour the orange juice into a measuring cup—you need ½ cup for the dressing. If you are short, squeeze the remaining orange until you have ½ cup. Whisk the yogurt and honey into the orange juice until smooth and pour it over the fruit. Cover with plastic wrap and refrigerate for at least 2 hours to allow the flavors to blend.

3. Meanwhile, line a small baking sheet with parchment paper. Combine the pecans, maple syrup, and ginger in a small saucepan and heat over medium heat. Cook, stirring constantly, until the syrup is sizzling and begins to turn sticky and golden brown. Keep a close watch as the syrup can burn easily. When the syrup is very thick and dark, pour the nuts out onto the lined baking sheet, separate with a fork, and let cool completely.

4. Cut the reserved orange peel into four ½-inch by 2-inch strips. To serve, divide the fruit salad among 4 serving bowls and top each with a few glazed pecans. Garnish each bowl with a twisted orange peel and serve immediately.

Oranges are famous for their high vitamin C content, one of the most powerful antioxidants and a well-known immune system support. This delicious citrus fruit also has a wide array of phytonutrients like flavanones, anthocyanins, and polyphenols. These antioxidant nutrients help protect you from the ravages of free radicals, thus protecting cells and DNA from the mutations that cause cancer. Vitamin C also supports the cardiovascular system, preventing the oxidation and hardening of cholesterol, risk factors in stroke and heart attack.

GRAPEFRUIT SALAD

BENEFITS: HEART + IMMUNITY + ANTI-INFLAMMATION + DIGESTION + GOOD MOOD

This is a very pretty fruit salad recipe that I picked up on my travels to the East Coast. Grapefruits have so many benefits! Extremely high in vitamin C, grapefruit helps support the immune system. It contains natural salicylic acid, which helps with arthritis, and is full of free-radical-fighting phytonutrients like limonoids and lycopene, which help prevent aging and defend against cancer. Additionally, grapefruit can lower cholesterol. Traditional Chinese medicine finds them to be a great aid in digestion. The dark red skin of the cranberries contains flavonoids that are powerful antioxidants and have bacteria-fighting properties. One warning: eating grapefruit is usually discouraged for people taking certain medications, as it can interfere with blood pressure and heart medications.

MAKES ABOUT 3 CUPS OR 4 SERVINGS

2 medium Ruby Red grapefruits, peeled
½ cup honey
¼ cup orange marmalade
1 cup fresh cranberries
2 medium bananas or 1 large banana

1. Using a sharp knife, section the grapefruit over a bowl, saving the juice and transferring the segments to another bowl. Pour the juice into a measuring cup and add enough water to the juice to measure ½ cup.

2. Put the juice mixture, honey, and marmalade into a small saucepan and bring to a boil, stirring to dissolve. Reduce the heat to medium-low, add the cranberries, and cook, stirring, until the cranberry skins pop, about 5 minutes. Remove from the heat and let cool.

3. Pour the cooled cranberry mixture over the grapefruit sections and refrigerate until ready to serve.

4. Just before serving, slice the bananas and stir into the chilled grapefruit mixture. Serve immediately.

The **banana** in this recipe helps balance out the tartness of the grapefruit, but anytime is a good time to indulge in this potassium-packed snack. Potassium is an essential mineral for maintaining normal blood pressure and heart function. In addition, bananas have long been recognized for their antacid effects, which protect against stomach ulcers. Very rich in B_6, bananas may help boost your mood, too!

MOUTHWATERING MELON DELIGHT

BENEFITS: HEART + IMMUNITY + BRAIN & VISION

Nothing says summer like a juicy, cooling watermelon! My mother used to make this for my brother and me during very hot summers in Asia, and it would cool us down immediately. Watermelon is an excellent source of the antioxidant lycopene, which has been associated with a reduced incidence of cancer, cardiovascular disease, and macular degeneration. It is also filled with vitamins A and C, making it good for your vision, and it contains the amino acid arginine, which helps lower blood pressure through its production of nitric oxide.

SERVES 4

1 cup chopped watermelon

¼ cup crumbled goat's milk feta cheese

1 small red onion, thinly sliced

¼ cup chopped fresh mint

Honey, for garnish

Combine the melon, cheese, onion, and mint in a serving bowl and mix gently. Drizzle a little honey over the top for a touch of added sweetness and serve immediately.

Mint pairs perfectly with many summer salads. Considered one of the most versatile herbs in traditional Chinese medicine, mint is known to relax the intestines, settle the stomach, and alleviate gas. Additionally, mint is rich in antioxidants that support good vision, and it cleanses your liver, helping eliminate harmful toxins from your body. Sprinkle mint on your food for flavor or steep in tea and drink thirty minutes after mealtimes for untroubled digestion.

COOL AND CRUNCHY SALAD

BENEFITS: HEART + IMMUNITY + ANTI-INFLAMMATION + DIGESTION + ANTI-AGING BEAUTY

This is a classic Middle Eastern recipe that is very cooling in the hot months, due in large part to the main ingredient. Cucumbers are a very popular vegetable, widely cultivated and used by many cultures. High in vitamin C and beta-carotene, cucumbers have anti-inflammatory properties and also anti-cancer properties, thanks to the lignans they possess. Radishes are high in fiber, which is particularly helpful with keeping digestion on track and fighting colon cancer. When paired with sunflower seeds, the complex carbohydrates of the vegetables are balanced out by the healthy fat and protein of the seeds. With veggie salads, you always want to achieve a nutritional harmony by adding beans, legumes, nuts, or seeds.

SERVES 4

1   chilled English cucumber, diced
4   small radishes, sliced
½   cup lowfat, unsweetened yogurt
2   tablespoons freshly squeezed
    lemon juice
1   tablespoon extra-virgin olive oil
1   teaspoon sunflower seeds,
    toasted and cooled
2   tablespoons mint, chopped

Combine the cucumber and radishes in a bowl. In a separate bowl, whisk the yogurt, lemon juice, and olive oil until combined and creamy. Add the dressing to the cucumbers and radishes and mix well. Sprinkle the toasted sunflower seeds and mint over the top of the salad for an aromatic and nutty crunch! Serve immediately.

It is no coincidence that one could be "cool as a **cucumber**." Cooling in nature, traditional Chinese medicine considers cucumber helpful for quenching thirst, relieving irritability, and promoting diuresis. As a natural diuretic, cucumber will help hydrate and lower the pressure in the arteries. It is also helpful for reducing inflammation in the body and has incredible anti-cancer properties. Cucumber's content of silica gives it the ability to soothe skin irritation and reduce swelling—so a slice on a bug bite can help minimize swelling. The cucumber is excellent in salads, as a snack alone, or pickled.

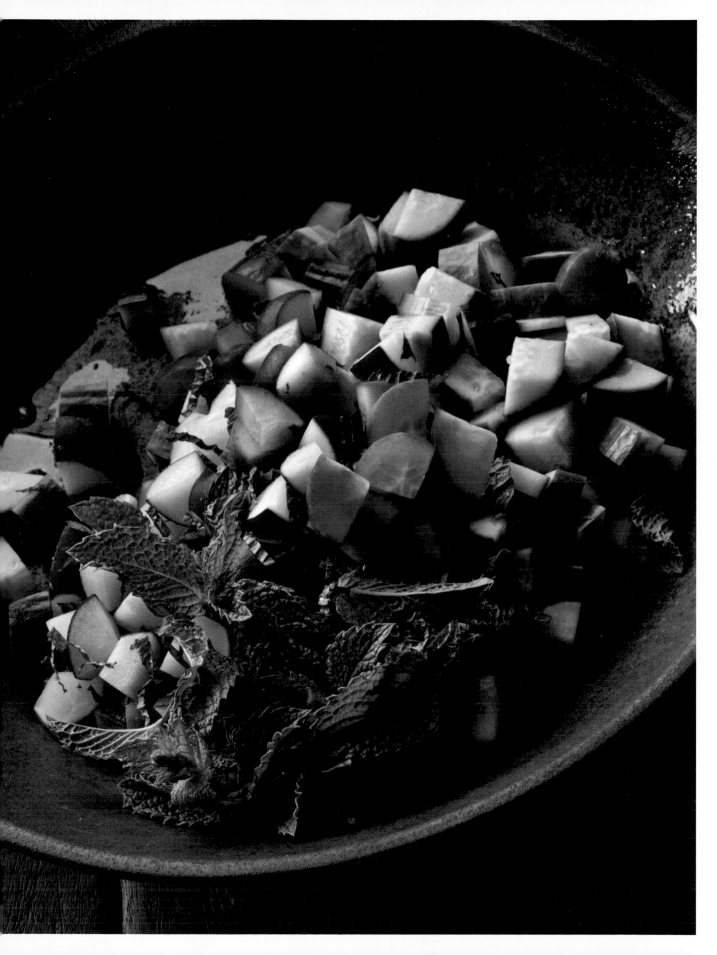

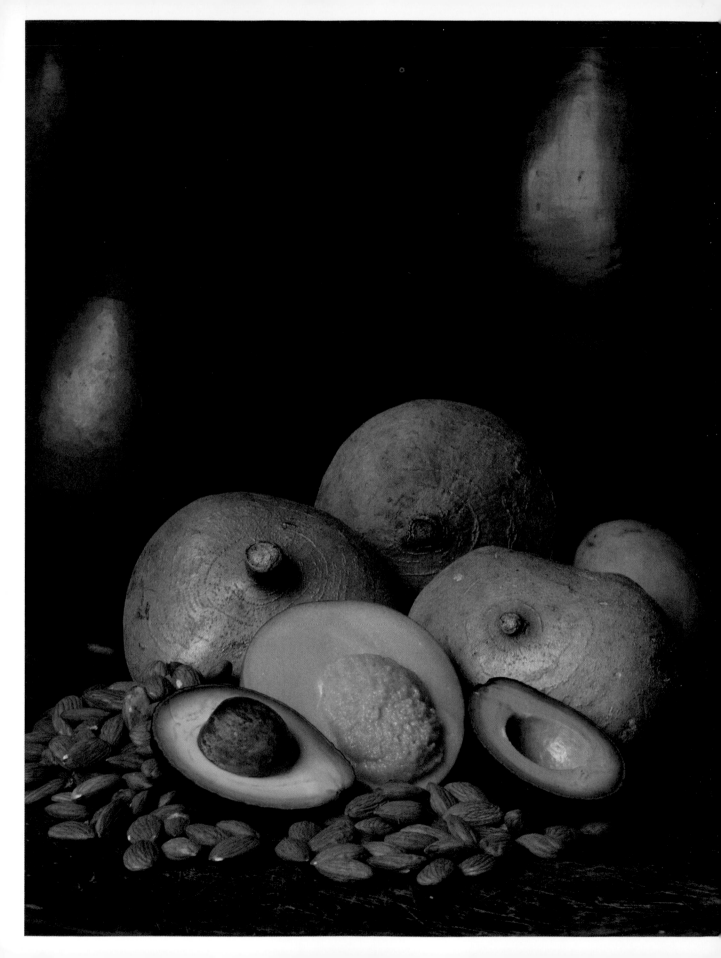

MANGO-AVOCADO SALAD

BENEFITS: HEART + ANTI-INFLAMMATION + METABOLISM + DIGESTION

A friend of mine from Peru grew up eating this salad recipe, which his grandmother used to make. His grandma lived to 104, so you can count this among one of the great tried-and-true longevity dishes and summertime favorites! Mango and avocados, very abundant in that part of the world, have many health benefits.

SERVES 4

1 large mango, peeled, pitted, and diced

1 large avocado, peeled, pitted, and diced

1 cup peeled and diced jicama

2 tablespoons chopped, toasted almonds

1 tablespoon dried cranberries

1 tablespoon freshly squeezed lemon juice

1 tablespoon extra-virgin olive oil

Toss the mango, avocado, jicama, almonds, and cranberries together in a medium bowl. Drizzle the lemon juice and olive oil over the fruit, toss gently to combine, and serve immediately.

Originally from Asia, **mangoes** were brought to South America in the fifteenth century. According to traditional Chinese medicine, the mango regenerates the body's fluids, stops coughs, and strengthens digestion. Indeed, they are especially rich in digestive enzymes and help detoxify the body. Mangoes also help strengthen the metabolism's function, which encourages weight loss and benefits cardiovascular health, helping to prevent high cholesterol, high blood pressure, and insulin resistance. Mangoes have been found to have incredible anti-inflammatory properties, hormone-regulating vitamin E, blood-building iron, and bone-strengthening minerals.

EDAMAME, SEAWEED, AND TOFU SALAD

BENEFITS: HEART + IMMUNITY + ANTI-INFLAMMATION

I received this recipe from a Japanese doctor, who is also a nutritionist. He came across this recipe in a traditional Japanese cookbook, and began recommending it to his patients because it was full of so many health benefits. It is a light, low-calorie salad, yet highly nutritious. The seaweed helps reduce inflammation and is an important source of trace minerals. The real star of this salad is the edamame, which is filled with protein and cholesterol-lowering properties, and it has also been found to help prevent breast and prostate cancer.

SERVES 4

DRESSING

⅓ cup rice vinegar
1½ tablespoons walnut oil
1½ teaspoons low-sodium soy sauce
1 teaspoon grated fresh ginger
½ teaspoon toasted sesame oil
  Small pinch cayenne pepper

SALAD

1 pound extra-firm tofu, cubed
½ small daikon radish, peeled and sliced into matchsticks
¼ ounce wakame seaweed, soaked in water for 1 hour
1½ teaspoons sesame seeds
2 cups frozen shelled edamame, thawed, rinsed, and patted dry
1 tablespoon chopped fresh cilantro

1. To make the dressing, in a large bowl, whisk the vinegar, walnut oil, soy sauce, ginger, sesame oil, and cayenne together until well combined. Gently fold in the tofu and radish until coated and set aside to marinate for 30 minutes.

2. Meawhile, bring a small saucepan of water to a boil and add the seaweed; boil for 15 minutes, until soft, and drain well. Put the sesame seeds in a small, dry skillet over medium-low heat and toast, swirling the pan, for about 3 minutes, or until golden and fragrant. Pour the seeds out onto a plate and cool.

3. Remove the tofu from the marinade and set aside on a plate. Add the drained seaweed and edamame to the dressing and toss well to combine. Gently fold the tofu back into the salad until evenly combined and transfer it to a serving plate.

4. Sprinkle the toasted sesame seeds over the top, garnish with chopped cilantro, and serve immediately.

Often found floating in miso soup, **wakame** looks like slippery spinach, but as you see here, it can also easily become a salad. It is a diuretic, which means it helps reduce the amount of water in the body. Because it prevents bloating and is packed with osteoporosis-preventing calcium and magnesium, wakame is sometimes referred to as the "women's seaweed." But the wakame benefits don't end there—this seaweed is also high in important trace minerals and is one of the few non-animal sources of vitamin B_{12}.

WARM COD SALAD

BENEFITS: HEART + BRAIN & VISION + GOOD MOOD

I had a patient from Norway who used to travel there often to see her relatives. She shared this recipe with me, and relished eating this family favorite because it had been a part of her Norwegian background for as long as she could remember. Her grandparents and great-grandparents lived into their nineties. Cod, like most other fish, has many cardiovascular benefits because it is such an excellent source of omega-3 fatty acids. When compared to most other forms of protein, fish is much easier to digest—helping you to really take advantage of the wonderful nutrients.

SERVES 4

1 (1-pound) skinless, boneless cod fillet
2 tablespoons coarse sea salt
1 cucumber, peeled and diced
10 cherry tomatoes, halved
1 avocado, peeled, pitted, and cubed
2 tablespoons freshly squeezed lime juice
5 tablespoons olive oil, divided
1 head butter lettuce, chopped
2 shallots, minced

1. Put the cod in a dish and rub the entire surface with the sea salt; refrigerate for 2 hours.

2. When ready to cook the fish, in a small bowl, gently toss the cucumbers, tomatoes, and avocado until combined. Drizzle the lime juice and 3 tablespoons of the olive oil over the vegetables and toss lightly to coat. Divide the lettuce among 4 serving plates and evenly distribute the cucumber mixture over the top of each plate of greens. Set aside while you cook the fish.

3. Rinse the cod fillet well under cold running water and pat very dry with a paper towel. Cut the fish into 1-inch chunks. Heat the remaining oil in a large nonstick skillet over medium-high heat. Add the cod and shallots and cook, turning and stirring frequently, until the fish is turning golden and is cooked through, 2 to 3 minutes.

4. Remove the fish from the heat and divide it evenly among the 4 salads. Serve immediately while warm.

Cod, like most fish, also has B vitamins, such as B_{12} and B_6, which fight against inflammation in blood vessels. Numerous studies show that people who eat a lot of fish—especially cold-water fish like cod—have less risk of heart attack, because the omega-3 fatty acids DHA and EPA are good for controlling blood pressure and helping to prevent blood clots. These fatty acids also help support eye health, boost brain health, and can even help elevate your mood. People who eat fish generally have higher IQs and lower rates of dementia; it may even protect against Alzheimer's. This tasty white, mild-flavored fish is available year-round. It is a good idea to get to know your local fishmonger so that you can get answers to any questions you may have about freshness and sustainability of their source.

SALMON LEEK SALAD WITH GINGER-MISO DRESSING

BENEFITS: HEART + IMMUNITY + ANTI-INFLAMMATION

My lovely wife adapted this dish from a Canadian friend of hers, who said this recipe had been in her family for some time. Her friend's family was from British Columbia, a place where salmon is abundant. My wife added an Asian flair with the ginger-miso dressing. Salmon has so many health benefits with its omega-3s, especially when combined with the leek, which is good for circulation.

SERVES 4

4   (6-ounce) boneless, skinless salmon fillets
20 thin slices fresh peeled ginger
    Salt
6   small leeks, trimmed and cut into ¼-inch slices
    Lettuce leaves, for serving

GINGER-MISO DRESSING
½   cup rice vinegar
¼   cup miso paste
1   teaspoon ground ginger

1. Preheat the oven to 325°F. Place a large sheet of parchment paper, large enough to loosely tent around all 4 pieces of salmon, on a baking pan. Rub the salmon pieces with a slice of ginger and season them to taste with salt. Place the salmon fillets in the center of the parchment paper on the pan and cover them with the ginger slices and leeks. Bring up the sides of paper, folding the top and sides to make a tent, enclosing the salmon completely. Bake until the salmon is cooked through, about 30 minutes.

2. Meanwhile, heat the vinegar in a small saucepan over low heat until warm. Add the miso paste and ground ginger, whisking until dissolved. Remove from heat.

3. Line 4 serving plates with lettuce leaves. Take the salmon out of the oven and carefully remove the leeks and ginger pieces from the salmon. Divide and arrange the leeks on top of the lettuce and top each plate with a salmon fillet. Pour the dressing over the salmon and garnish with the cooked ginger slices. Serve warm or cold.

Considered a warming food, **leeks** perk up the immune system with their rich sources of vitamin C, potassium, chromium, and selenium. Additionally, they contain volatile oils that are antimicrobial and help stimulate immunity. Leeks guard you from diseases like diabetes, arthritis, heart diseases, and certain forms of cancer.

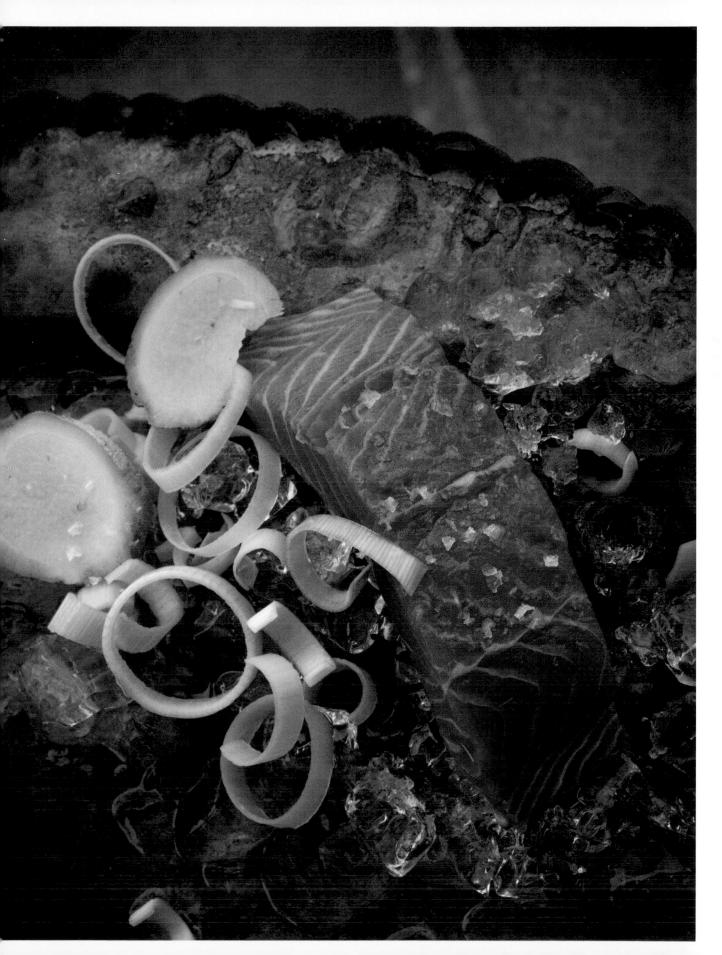

SMALL DISHES

I call this section "Small Dishes" because the portions are a bit smaller than what we have grown accustomed to in the U.S. I wanted to tap into the European idea of eating smaller portions of high-quality food, which is good for your heart, great for your digestion, and helpful with weight loss. Many European cultures eat a mid-afternoon meal. Take, for instance, the English mid-afternoon high tea. They give themselves a little snack and then don't feel so drained in the afternoon or so famished by dinnertime. The real inspiration for this section and the smaller portions in this book are Spanish *tapas*, a variety of snacks that you eat slowly as you make conversation with others. While we will not excessively partake in the requisite alcoholic drink that usually accompanies *tapas*, the recipes in this section offer plenty of snack-size items that are easy to prepare, mouthwateringly tasty, and incredibly healing.

More than half of these recipes are vegetarian, and will teach you how you can easily make a delicious meal that does not rely on the usual entrée centerpiece of meat with a few afterthought sides. The majority of the non-vegetarian recipes feature fish, because it is full of healthy fats that support your heart and brain health, as well as being the animal product most frequently eaten by centenarians. Cheers to your health and longevity!

GRILLED PORTOBELLO MUSHROOMS WITH GOAT FETA

BENEFITS: IMMUNITY

I came across this classic Italian recipe at a friend's summer barbecue, and the combination is just right for longevity. Goat's milk or sheep's milk dairy is high in protein and is much easier to digest than cow's milk. The portobellos, like all mushrooms, benefit the immune system. The feta cheese flavors combine so well with the portobello that you practically don't have to season this dish!

SERVES 4

4   medium portobello mushrooms, washed and patted dry
½   cup olive oil, plus more for garnish
2   tablespoons freshly squeezed lemon juice
2   cloves garlic, crushed
1   tablespoon fresh oregano leaves
1   tablespoon fresh mint leaves
1   red chili, seeded and minced
½   cup crumbled goat's milk feta cheese
1   handful flat-leaf parsley, chopped, for garnish

1. Place the mushrooms on a baking sheet. Put the olive oil, lemon juice, garlic, oregano, mint, and red chili into a blender or food processor and pulse until it forms a thick sauce. Brush the sauce on both sides of the mushrooms.

2. Preheat a stovetop grill pan over medium-high heat. When it starts to smoke, grill the mushrooms, turning once, until grill marks appear and the mushroom is softened and releasing juice, about 10 minutes.

3. Transfer the mushrooms to a serving platter, scatter the cheese over the warm mushrooms, drizzle a little oil over each, garnish with parsley, and serve immediately.

I usually don't recommend **grilling** because people often burn their food on the grill, creating carcinogens that are very bad for you. In this case, the mushrooms are placed on a grill pan and not directly on the grill, which gives you the flavor without the char. Make sure you always monitor your food on the grill to be sure it isn't burning, and keep grilling in general to a minimum, no more than once a week.

STUFFED CUCUMBER CUPS WITH SHIITAKE MUSHROOMS AND LOTUS ROOT

BENEFITS: IMMUNITY + CLEANSING + ANTI-AGING BEAUTY

This recipe was collected during my interviews with centenarians in China. The shiitake mushroom is known to boost the immune system while the lotus root promotes detoxification. These two ingredients together make a formidable food combination to boost immunity and provide prevention and support of cancer.

SERVES 4 TO 6

2   fresh lotus roots, peeled and thinly sliced crosswise
4   thin English cucumbers
10 dried shiitake mushrooms, soaked in warm water for 1 hour
2   tablespoons sesame oil, plus more as needed
4   scallions, finely chopped
4   shallots, finely chopped
3   red chilies, seeded and finely chopped
1   teaspoon salt

1. Preheat the oven to 375°F. Spread the lotus root out on a baking sheet and bake for 20 minutes. Remove and set aside several pieces for garnish. Chop the remaining lotus root into small chunks.

2. Wash the cucumbers thoroughly and pat them dry with a paper towel. Cut the ends off the cucumbers and slice them into chunks about 1½ inches thick. Stand the slices upright and scoop out the center of each cucumber piece with a melon baller or teaspoon, leaving a base in the bottom of each cup.

3. Drain the mushrooms and remove and discard the stems. Heat the oil in a wok over medium-high heat. Add the mushrooms and stir-fry until softened, about 5 minutes. Remove the wok from the heat, transfer the mushrooms to a cutting board, and cool briefly; coarsely chop them.

4. Heat the wok again over medium heat and add the scallions, shallots, and red chilies; stir-fry for 5 minutes. Add the chopped lotus root, mushrooms, and salt to the wok and stir-fry for another 2 to 3 minutes. Transfer the vegetables to a bowl and let cool.

5. Put the garnishing slices of lotus root into the wok and stir-fry until slightly brown, adding a little oil if necessary to keep them from sticking. Take care not to break them. Remove promptly.

6. Fill the cucumber cups with the cooled filling. Garnish with the slices of lotus root and serve immediately.

Considered an herb by traditional Chinese medicine, the **lotus root** is an Asian vegetable that is similar in shape to a long squash. It is a gentle diuretic, which is helpful for kidney support and ridding the body of excess water. High in fiber and packed with many significant vitamins and minerals, lotus root is notable for its high content of vitamin C. Vitamin C is essential for collagen synthesis in the body and helps boost immunity and remove cancer-causing free radicals. Lotus root can be found in Asian markets and online.

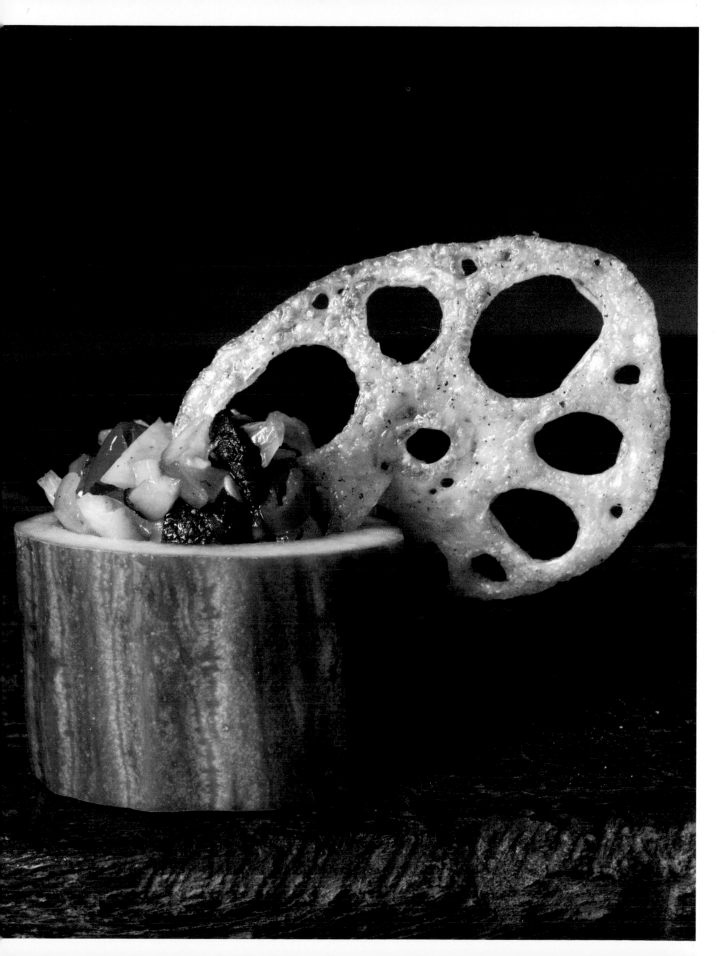

BRAISED CHICORY WITH RED WINE VINEGAR

BENEFITS: HEART

Chicory is not usually eaten as a vegetable in the U.S., except for in the South. A patient of mine from Georgia shared this simple family dish of braised chicory that he and his long-living parents have been eating regularly for years. They obviously didn't subscribe to the typical Southern diet! The chicory combined with the vinegar will not only satisfy your taste buds but will also keep your heart strong and healthy.

SERVES 4

1   tablespoon olive oil
8   chicory heads, trimmed
⅓   cup chicken or vegetable stock
2   teaspoons red wine vinegar
1   teaspoon maple syrup
2   tablespoons walnut oil
1   tablespoon finely chopped
     chives, for garnish

1. Heat the olive oil in a large skillet over medium heat. Add the chicory and cook, turning frequently, until lightly browned on all sides. Add the stock, vinegar, and maple syrup and cook until it begins to boil. Reduce the heat to low, cover, and cook for 30 minutes, or until the chicory is tender and a knife inserted into the cores meets little resistance.

2. Remove the lid and continue simmering until the liquid has nearly evaporated, 10 to 15 minutes more. Transfer the chicory to 4 serving bowls, drizzle some walnut oil over each, garnish with the chives, and serve immediately.

A vegetable commonly eaten in Asia and parts of Europe, **chicory** is most commonly used in the U.S. as a coffee substitute—but it is very tasty when braised as a vegetable. Considered a health tonic in traditional Chinese medicine, chicory contains a compound called inulin that has been found useful in preventing and treating congestive heart failure. Additionally, research has found that chicory can slow a rapid heartbeat, help lower cholesterol, and slow the progression of hardening of the arteries.

SEAWEED AND VEGETABLE MEDLEY

BENEFITS: HEART + ANTI-INFLAMMATION + METABOLISM + CLEANSING

This is another recipe that comes from Chinese centenarians I interviewed. Seaweed has more concentrated nutrition than vegetables grown on land and has long been considered to possess powers to prolong life, prevent disease, and impart beauty and health. For thousands of years, this mineral-rich vegetable has been a staple in Asian diets. Combined with the antioxidant-rich vegetables, this is one longevity recipe to celebrate!

SERVES 4

1 (15-inch) piece kombu seaweed
10 small dried Chinese mushrooms
1 small carrot, cut into 2-inch pieces, and thinly sliced lengthwise
1 cup snow peas, trimmed (halved crosswise if large)
6 stalks asparagus, trimmed and cut into 2-inch pieces
1 medium green bell pepper, seeded and cut into bite-size pieces
1 tablespoon grapeseed oil
   Sea salt and freshly ground pepper

1. In two separate bowls, soak the kombu and mushrooms in warm water until softened. Drain the kombu and cut it into 1-inch pieces. Strain the mushrooms, reserving the soaking water. Remove the mushroom stems and discard; quarter the caps.

2. Put the mushroom soaking water into a medium saucepan over medium-low heat. Add the kombu and mushrooms, cover, and cook until very tender, adding water if the pan dries out. Increase the heat to medium, add the carrot, cover, and continue cooking for 3 minutes. Add the snow peas, asparagus, and pepper, increase the heat to high, cover, and cook for 3 minutes more.

3. Remove the pan from the heat, stir in the oil, season with salt and pepper to taste, and mix until combined. Serve the medley hot.

With its powerful trace minerals, **kombu** aids your body in detoxification. It comes in long, thick brown strips and is valuable for its high content of iodine, which is needed to produce two important thyroid hormones that control the metabolism. Our bodies don't make iodine, so we have to get it through food. Many people are thyroid deficient—kombu can come to the rescue with its iodine content. Also, there is a pigment in kombu called fucoxanthin, which may boost production of a protein involved in fat metabolism. You can find kombu in many health-food stores, Asian markets, and online.

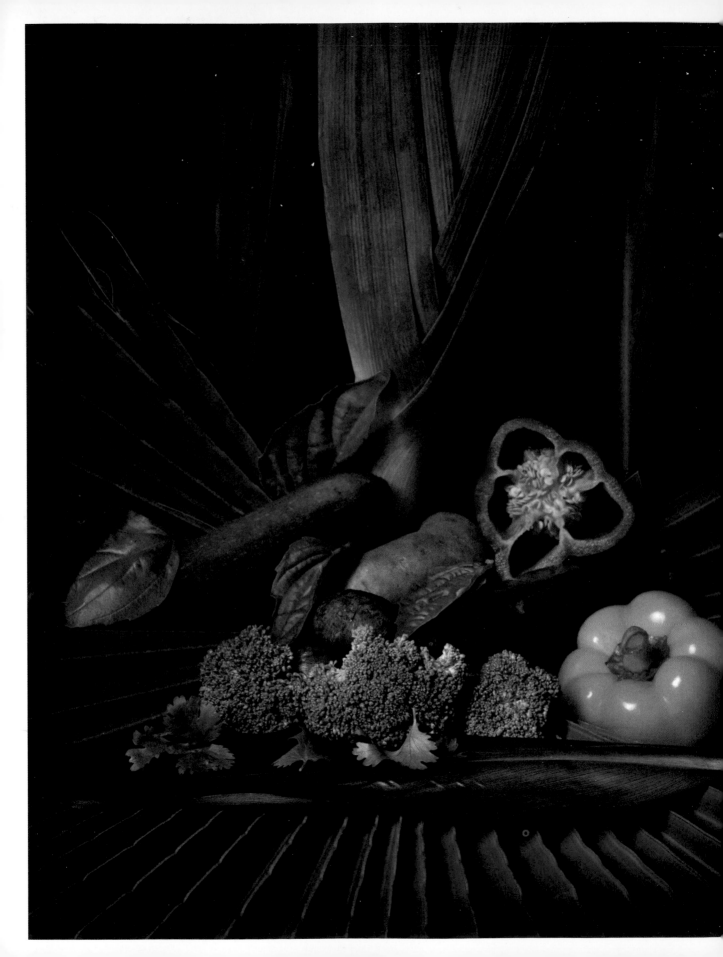

BROCCOLI STIR-FRY WITH YAM NOODLES

BENEFITS: IMMUNITY + ANTI-INFLAMMATION + BRAIN & VISION

This dish is a staple of the Japanese centenarian diet. Anti-cancerous, anti-inflammatory, and rich in antioxidants, broccoli is a cruciferous vegetable that helps boost immunity, brain health, and vision health, among many other beneficial talents. Combined with the other vegetables, herbs, and yam noodles, this tasty dish is incredibly high in fiber and antioxidants.

SERVES 4

1 (1-pound) package yam noodles
1 tablespoon walnut or peanut oil
2 cloves garlic, thinly sliced
2 leeks, trimmed and cut diagonally
   into ⅛-inch thick slices
2 cups broccoli florets
2 carrots, thinly sliced
1 cup half-moon zucchini slices
¼ cup water or vegetable broth
5 white button mushrooms, sliced
1 red bell pepper, cored, seeded,
   and cut lengthwise into thin strips
1 tablespoon chopped fresh basil
1 tablespoon chopped fresh cilantro
1 tablespoon tamari

1. Bring a saucepan of water to a boil and cook the yam noodles according to the package instructions, rinse under cold water, and reserve. Fill the pan with water again and bring to a boil.

2. Heat the oil in a wok or large skillet over medium-high heat. Add the garlic and leeks and sauté until crisp-tender, 3 to 4 minutes. Add the broccoli, carrots, zucchini, and water or broth. Cover the pan and cook, stirring frequently, for 5 minutes. Add the mushrooms and red bell pepper and continue cooking, stirring constantly, for 5 minutes. Add the basil, cilantro, and tamari. Stir well and remove from the heat.

3. Drop the cooked yam noodles into the boiling water for 10 seconds to reheat. Drain in a colander and shake well. Divide the warm noodles among 4 serving plates and ladle the vegetable stir-fry over each plate. Serve immediately.

High in fiber, **yam noodles** are starchy, but not high on the glycemic index—so the body doesn't have the same sugar reaction it would have to wheat pasta. Yams in general have many benefits, including that they contain nutrients that help them balance blood sugar, making them good for those who suffer from blood sugar imbalance, including diabetics. Yams also contain a protein that helps lower high blood pressure. In traditional Chinese medicine, the yam is considered a digestive and kidney tonic. You can find fresh yam noodles in Asian markets or in the refrigerated section of many health-food stores.

ALMOND AND VEGGIE STIR-FRY

BENEFITS: HEART + IMMUNITY + ANTI-AGING BEAUTY

This tasty stir-fry was shared with me by a patient from Hong Kong. She remembered this as the dish that got her to eat vegetables when she was very young and didn't care for them. The texture and taste of the extremely beneficial almonds cast the vegetables in a delicious light. Try this one out on any friends or family you know who don't want to eat their veggies!

SERVES 4

2   small yams or sweet potatoes, cut into bite-size pieces
1   small head cauliflower, cut into bite-size pieces
2   leeks or 1 medium onion, sliced
1   summer squash, stemmed and cut into bite-size pieces
1   handful green beans, cut into bite-size pieces
1   cup white button mushrooms, quartered
4   teaspoons toasted sesame oil
½   cup sliced almonds
2   tablespoons arrowroot powder
2   tablespoons water
    Salt and freshly ground black pepper
    Toasted sesame seeds, for garnish

1. Put the yams, cauliflower, leeks, squash, green beans, and mushrooms into a large, deep skillet and pour in just enough water to cover the bottom of the pan. Bring to a boil, reduce the heat to medium-low, cover, and cook until the vegetables are just tender, about 10 minutes.

2. Meanwhile, put 2 teaspoons of the oil into a small skillet over medium-low heat. Add the almonds and cook, stirring, until light golden brown. Remove from the heat.

3. In a small bowl, whisk the arrowroot powder with 2 tablespoons water until dissolved. Remove the lid from the vegetables and stir in the arrowroot mixture. Season the vegetables with salt and pepper to taste, and cook until the liquid thickens, 1 to 2 minutes. Add the toasted almonds and remaining sesame oil to the vegetables and stir well to combine. Remove from the heat, garnish with sesame seeds, and serve immediately.

High in healthy monounsaturated fats, **almonds** have been linked with lower LDL cholesterol levels and reduced risk of heart disease by many studies. Almonds are also high in vitamin E, which acts as an antioxidant and also has heart-protective properties. In addition, a quarter-cup of almonds contains one quarter of your daily value for magnesium, an essential mineral that benefits heart function, aids in bone growth, and may protect skin from UV damage. According to studies, the healthy fats in almonds may even be able to help you lose weight.

BROWN RICE WITH PINE NUTS

BENEFITS: HEART + IMMUNITY + BRAIN & VISION + ANTI-AGING BEAUTY

While interviewing a 101-year-old man from Kunming, China, I learned about this simple, tasty recipe. He liked to cook nuts and seeds with his rice, which I found delicious. This recipe was one of my favorites of his nut-rice combinations. Not only does it add a deliciously nutty flavor and texture to the brown rice, but pine nuts are chock-full of nutrients—essential fatty acids, anti-oxidants like pycnogenol, and protein. This dish could easily serve as a quick meal on the go or a wonderful complement to any main course.

SERVES 4

2 cups whole-grain brown rice
½ cup pine nuts, toasted
⅓ cup minced fresh dill, optional

Prepare the rice according to the package directions. While still warm, toss the rice with the pine nuts and dill in a serving bowl. Serve warm or at room temperature.

Pine nuts are not actually nuts at all, but the edible seeds of pinecones. They are very beneficial for heart health because, like nuts, they are high in monounsaturated fats. In addition, the potent antioxidant called pycnogenol protects the vascular endothelial cells (which make up the lining of the heart and blood vessels) from free radical damage. Pycnogenol also helps protect the brain from free radicals, works as an anti-inflammatory, and helps preserve skin structure. Pine nuts can go rancid quickly, but you can extend their life by keeping them in the refrigerator.

VEGETABLE ALMOND PIE

BENEFITS: IMMUNITY + ANTI-INFLAMMATION + BRAIN & VISION

This dish is totally satisfying, high in fiber, and provides all your recommended daily portions of vegetables in one complete meal. It is a great way to get children who don't like vegetables to eat them. In fact, this is a recipe my mother used to make for my brother and me, and we loved it so much, we used to fight over it! When we were growing up, she used to juice vegetables a lot, and after juicing, she would have a pile of leftover pulp. Instead of tossing it, she would bake it in a pie, which is how this recipe came about. You can do the same, and feel free to vary the vegetables to your taste.

SERVES 4

CRUST

1   cup brown rice flour, plus more for rolling
2   tablespoons avocado oil
¼   cup sesame seeds
2   tablespoons sesame tahini

FILLING

2   turnips, chopped
2   carrots, chopped
1   onion, minced
2   cloves garlic, minced
1   head purple cabbage, chopped
1   1-inch piece fresh ginger, peeled and finely minced
3   tablespoons sesame oil
¼   cup peanut butter
1   tablespoon honey
1   tablespoon vinegar
    Sea salt
3   tablespoons arrowroot powder
1½ cups water
½   cup sliced almonds

1. Preheat the oven to 375°F. To make the crust, put the flour, oil, sesame seeds, and tahini into a mixing bowl and mix by hand until a soft dough forms. Lightly flour a work surface and press or roll the crust into a rough 14-inch circle. Transfer the dough to a deep 10-inch pie plate and press the dough evenly into it. Fold the edges around the rim of the plate under to create a lip. Bake for 15 minutes.

2. To make the filling, put about ¼ cup water into a large saucepan and heat it over medium-high heat. When the water is bubbling, add the turnips, carrots, onion, garlic, cabbage, and ginger. Stir the vegetables, cover, and cook for 10 minutes. Make sure there is enough water in the pan to avoid burning the vegetables. Add the sesame oil, peanut butter, honey, vinegar, and salt to taste. Reduce the heat to low.

3. Dissolve the arrowroot powder in 1½ cups water and slowly stir into vegetables; cook until thickened. Pour the vegetable mixture into the pie crust, top with the almonds, and bake until the crust is golden brown and the filling is thick and bubbly, about 45 minutes.

4. Cool the pie on a rack for at least 30 minutes before slicing and serving.

The crust in this recipe is made with **sesame** goodness, thanks to its ¼ cup of seeds and tahini. Rich in antioxidant properties, sesame seeds add a delicious nutty flavor and crunch to your meals, while providing your body with crucial nutrients. One large handful (about ¼ cup) of sesame seeds gives you approximately 74 percent of the daily value for copper, 31 percent of magnesium, 35 percent of calcium, and about 30 percent of iron. In addition, sesame seeds are rich in zinc, which improves bone mineral density. Zinc is also a powerful immune booster and may potentially shorten the duration of colds.

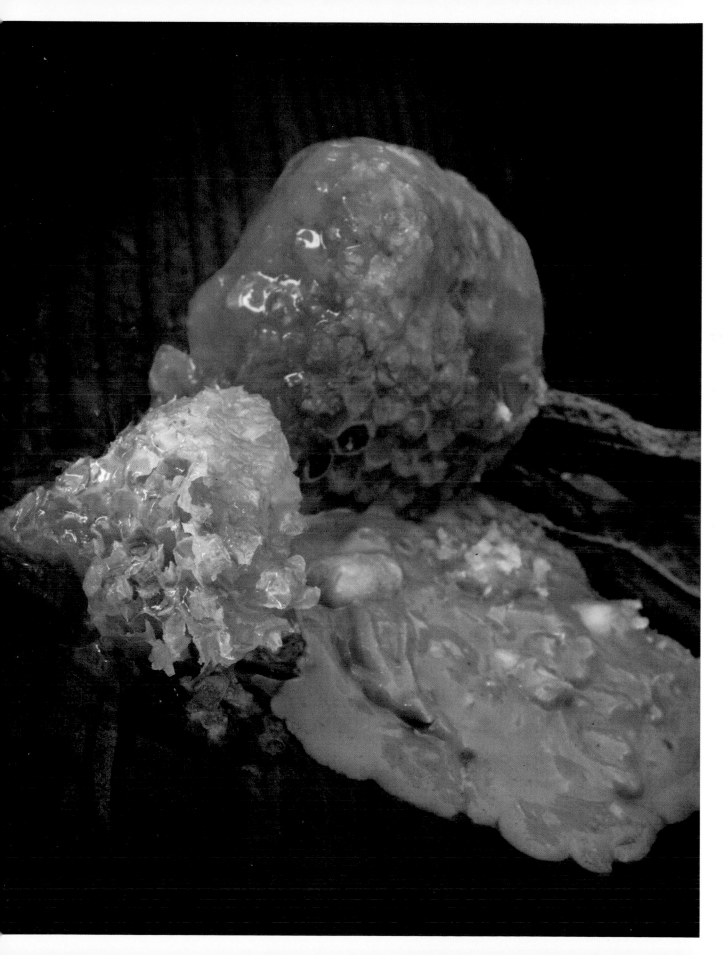

STUFFED PUMPKIN

BENEFITS: HEART + IMMUNITY + METABOLISM + BRAIN & VISION

This simple and easy-to-make recipe came from a patient of mine who claimed that it was her parents' favorite recipe. Both of her parents are still living and are in their nineties, so it must be a good match for longevity! I can see why: the pumpkin's rich content of vitamins like beta-carotene, sesame's supply of rich fatty acids and lignans, celery's support of strong bones, and onions for immune health make this dish deliciously healthy.

SERVES 4 TO 6

1   small pumpkin, about 4 pounds (small enough to fit inside a large Dutch oven with a lid)
    Vegetable oil
3   cups cooked brown rice
1   tablespoon toasted sesame seeds, crushed
3   stalks celery, chopped
1   onion, finely chopped
1   tablespoon chopped fresh parsley
1   teaspoon fresh thyme leaves
1   teaspoon chopped fresh sage
½   teaspoon chopped fresh rosemary
1   tablespoon tamari

1. Preheat the oven to 350°F. Grease a large Dutch oven with oil.

2. Wash the exterior of the pumpkin well. Cut off the top, clean out the seeds and membranes, and discard. Rub the exterior of the pumpkin with oil and put it into the Dutch oven. Put the pumpkin lid on and then check to see if the Dutch oven lid fits; trim or remove the pumpkin stem if necessary.

3. In a large bowl, stir the rice, sesame seeds, celery, onion, parsley, thyme, sage, rosemary, and tamari together until well combined. Transfer the stuffing to the pumpkin cavity, replace the pumpkin top and cover with the lid. Bake for 1¼ to 1½ hours, until a fork easily pierces the pumpkin.

4. Remove from the oven, remove the lid, and let the pumpkin stand about 10 minutes. Carefully use two large spoons to transfer the pumpkin to a serving platter. Serve whole at the table for guests to help themselves to the softened pumpkin and stuffing.

As this recipe shows, **pumpkins** have more uses than just serving as jack-o'lanterns! Pumpkins are rich in potassium and a good source of iron, zinc, and fiber. The bright orange flesh is loaded with beta-carotene, which keeps your immune system strong, benefits vision, helps prevent heart disease, and may defend against cancer. The pumpkin is also the perfect fit for losing weight due to its incredibly low calorie count and high fiber content. The sweetest taste can be found in the small-size pumpkin varieties known as sugar pumpkin or pie pumpkin.

ROASTED CHESTNUTS AND WOOD EAR MUSHROOMS WITH BROWN RICE

BENEFITS: IMMUNITY + ANTI-INFLAMMATION

Another of my favorite mixed nut-rice combinations from Chinese centenarians, this unique recipe contains chestnut, considered a kidney tonic in Chinese medical nutrition, and is rich in B-complex like folate, vitamin C, and fiber. Do not be afraid of the wood ear mushroom! It is easier to come by than you might think, and has been found to possess incredible anti-cancer, anti-inflammatory, and antioxidant properties. Together, chestnut and wood ear mushroom form a powerful duo in this colorful and delicious dish.

SERVES 4

1   cup brown rice
1   cup dried whole chestnuts
    Grapeseed oil
5   dried shiitake mushrooms
3   pieces dried wood ear
    mushrooms
¼   cup peas, fresh or frozen
¼   cup corn kernels, fresh or frozen
¼   cup diced water chestnuts
2   teaspoons olive oil
    Sea salt and freshly ground black
    pepper

1. Soak the rice and chestnuts in a large bowl with 3 cups of water overnight (or in hot water for 1 hour).

2. Preheat the oven to 250°F. Separate the chestnuts from the rice and put them in a roasting pan. Drizzle some grapeseed oil over the chestnuts and roast them in the oven for 15 to 20 minutes, until soft. Set aside. Pour the rice and soaking water into a saucepan and bring to a boil over medium-high heat. Reduce the heat to medium-low, cover, and simmer for 45 minutes. Remove from the heat and set aside.

3. Meanwhile, soak the shiitake and wood ear mushrooms in water for 1 hour. Drain them, slice, and put into a saucepan with about ¼ cup of water. Bring the mushrooms to a simmer over medium heat, cover, and cook for 25 minutes, or until tender.

4. Add roasted chestnuts, peas, corn, and water chestnuts to the mushrooms and cook for another 5 minutes. Remove from the heat, stir in the olive oil, and season with salt and pepper to taste. Combine the chestnut mixture with the rice, stir well, and serve.

Unlike other nuts and seeds, **chestnuts** are fairly low in calories and fat, but still contain a wide array of beneficial vitamins and minerals. Very high in fiber, chestnuts can help lower cholesterol levels. Chestnuts' rich source of vitamin C protects against free radical damage and bolsters immunity. Of all the nuts, chestnuts contain one of the highest levels of folate. As a nut, it contains high levels of essential fatty acids, such as linoleic acid, which benefit heart health. Provided you aren't allergic, these crunchy treats will serve you and your longevity well.

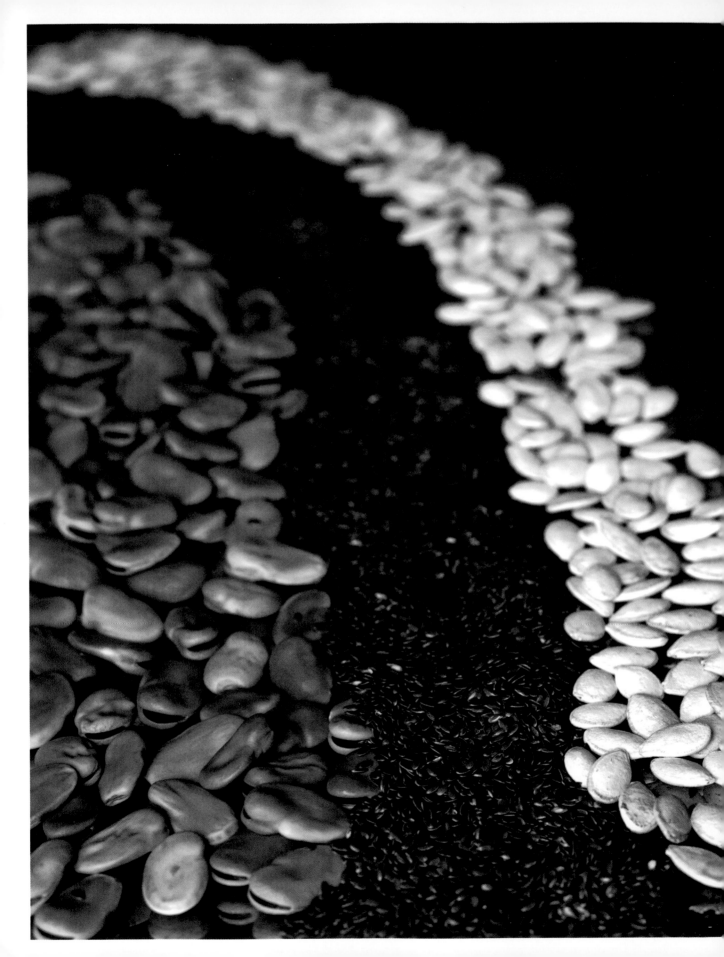

MILLET PILAF

BENEFITS: HEART + METABOLISM

Millet is an under-appreciated grain in America, but very popular with the centenarians of China. If you have never tried this little yellow grain, you are in for a treat! Millet is nutritionally richer than wheat and has the bonus of being gluten-free. This recipe is a popular one among many centenarians, which is not surprising, as it is a nice balance of nutrients and healthy oils with beneficial herbs and spices.

SERVES 4

1¼ cups vegetable stock
1   onion, chopped
1   clove garlic, minced
1   cinnamon stick
2   bay leaves
1   teaspoon ground cardamom
1   cup millet
¾   cup frozen peas, thawed
1   cup frozen fava beans, thawed
½   cup pumpkin seeds
2   tablespoons finely chopped fresh parsley
1   tablespoon finely chopped fresh mint

1. Heat ¼ cup of the vegetable stock in a large saucepan over medium heat. Add the onion and garlic and sauté for 4 to 5 minutes, or until softened. Add the cinnamon stick, bay leaves, and cardamom and cook for a few more minutes. Remove the cinnamon stick and bay leaves and discard. Stir in the millet and remaining vegetable stock and bring to a boil. Reduce the heat to medium-low, cover, and simmer for 20 minutes. Check occasionally and add water if the pan is dry.

2. Stir the peas and fava beans into the millet, cover, and cook for another 5 to 7 minutes. Uncover the pan and fluff the millet with a fork. Stir in the pumpkin seeds, parsley, and mint and transfer the millet to a serving bowl.

3. Serve warm or at room temperature.

Though technically a seed, **millet** is categorized as a grain from a culinary perspective. A good source of magnesium and fiber, millet can significantly lower the risk of cardiovascular disease, obesity, insulin resistance, and type 2 diabetes. Millet contains a phytonutrient called plant lignans, which may help protect against breast cancer and heart disease. All this, and gluten-free, too!

ROSEMARY MILLET WITH YELLOW SPLIT PEAS AND ZUCCHINI FLOWERS

BENEFITS: HEART + BRAIN & VISION + GOOD MOOD

A vendor at the farmer's market where I buy zucchini flowers shared this recipe with me. He alleged that it came from his grandmother who was almost ninety years of age. The nutritious millet is paired with yellow split peas, which are no longevity slouch! They contain high levels of tryptophan to help support healthy sleep and balanced moods. Dress it up with beautiful zucchini flowers and rosemary, which stimulates your brain's activity—and you've got a recipe that promotes happiness.

SERVES 4

1   cup millet
½   cup yellow split peas
½   cup corn kernels, fresh or
     frozen
2   teaspoons virgin coconut oil
     Sea salt and freshly ground
     black pepper
2   sprigs of fresh rosemary,
     leaves stripped and chopped
4 to 8 zucchini flowers

1. Put the millet and split peas into a saucepan, add 3½ cups water, and bring to a boil over medium-high heat. Reduce the heat to medium-low, cover, and simmer for 1 hour.

2. Stir the corn into the millet, cover, and continue cooking for an additional 30 minutes, adding a little water to the pan if necessary. When the split peas are tender, remove the pan from the heat, stir in the coconut oil, season with salt and pepper to taste, and mix well. Ladle the millet into bowls and garnish with rosemary and one or two zucchini flowers on top.

A member of the legume family, **split yellow peas** are simply peas that have been dried and split. They are high in protein, an excellent source of fiber, and have virtually no fat. Their high fiber content helps stabilize blood sugar levels, beneficial for those with insulin resistance and diabetes. Additionally, the yellow split pea also contains molybdenum, which effectively detoxifies sulfites for those who are sensitive to their presence in prepared food. When paired with a grain, as they are in this recipe with millet, they become a complete protein, essential for those who don't eat meat.

CURRY VEGETABLES WITH BROWN RICE

BENEFITS: HEART + ANTI-INFLAMMATION

More than twenty years ago, a swami from India shared this favorite recipe with me. Judging from his advanced age but amazingly fit physique, I am convinced that the combination of brown rice, tofu, and vegetables provided a balanced and nutritious meal for a vegetarian. And don't forget the health benefits of curry! This orangey spice blend contains turmeric and other spices that promote circulation, prevent blood clots, and decrease inflammation—all of which help protect you from heart disease.

SERVES 4

1   cup brown rice
1   medium potato, diced
1   medium carrot, diced
⅓   pound firm tofu, diced
⅓   cup peas, fresh or frozen
5   white button mushrooms, quartered
¼   green bell pepper, chopped
1   stalk celery, chopped
2   tablespoons cornstarch
1   tablespoon curry powder
½   cup water
1   teaspoon walnut oil
    Sea salt and freshly ground black pepper
    Fresh cilantro sprigs, for garnish

1. Place the rice in a saucepan with 2 cups of water and bring to a boil over medium-high heat. Reduce the heat to medium-low, cover, and simmer for 40 minutes. Set aside. The rice can also be cooked in a pressure cooker for 15 minutes.

2. Bring 2 cups of water to a boil in a large, deep skillet. Add the potato, cover, turn the heat to low, and cook for 10 minutes. Add the carrot and tofu and cook, covered, for another 10 minutes. Increase the heat to high and add the peas, mushrooms, green pepper and celery and cook for 2 minutes.

3. In a small bowl, stir the cornstarch and curry powder together and add the water; whisk until smooth. Pour the mixture slowly into the pan, stirring gently until thickened. Remove the curry from the heat, stir in the walnut oil, and season with salt and pepper to taste.

4. To serve, divide the brown rice among 4 plates and pour the curry vegetables over the rice. Garnish with the cilantro sprigs.

White rice begins as **brown rice**—but once the outer coating of rice bran is hulled off, not a lot of nutrients remain. Modern research has identified a bounty of nutrients—including over seventy antioxidants!—in the bran coating of brown rice, which are effective at lowering high blood sugar, making brown rice a good food for diabetics. The fiber content is also impressive, and helps protect against colon cancer and plaque build-up that narrows blood vessels. With all these benefits, it's not surprising that rural farmers in Asia, who eat less costly brown rice, live longer and develop fewer health issues than their city-dwelling counterparts, who eat mostly more expensive white rice.

QUINOA BROWN RICE SUSHI

BENEFITS: HEART + METABOLISM

My mother innovated constantly to satisfy her two sons' demanding palates, so she adapted quinoa with brown rice to make one of our all-time favorite foods: sushi. Once called "Inca Gold" due to its stamina-building properties, quinoa contains all the essential amino acids, rendering it a complete protein food. Its high manganese content supplies the body's production of superoxide dismutase, an enzyme that protects against free radical damage to your energy factory. Consider this an energizing longevity recipe!

SERVES 4

1	cup sticky brown rice
½	cup quinoa
8	ounces baked bean curd/tofu, cut into long thin strips
4 to 5	carrots, cut into matchsticks
4	nori seaweed sheets
2	pickled cucumbers (low-sodium), cut into matchsticks
2	avocados, peeled, pitted, and sliced
	Cilantro sprigs, for garnish
	Pickled ginger, for garnish

1. Place the rice, quinoa, and 3 cups water into a rice cooker and cook according to the manufacturer's instructions. (You can also cook the rice and quinoa in 3 cups water in a pressure cooker for 15 minutes).

2. Bring a saucepan of water to a boil and cook the carrots until softened, about 30 seconds. Drain and rinse them under cold water.

3. Unroll a bamboo sushi mat on a work surface and put a sheet of nori on it. Wet your hands and divide the rice into 4 equal portions. Divide one portion into 4 small, firm balls and press them evenly onto the nori, covering the entire sheet with a thin layer of grains. Evenly spread one-quarter of the bean curd, one-quarter of the carrots, one-quarter of the cucumbers, and one-quarter of the avocado in the center of the rice. Using the mat as a guide, roll the topped nori tightly and evenly into a sushi roll, wetting the edges of the nori sheet with water if necessary, so it sticks together at the seam. Repeat three more times with the remaining nori, rice, and vegetables.

4. Slice the rolls into 1½-inch-thick pieces with a sharp, wet knife and transfer them to a serving platter. Garnish with cilantro and pickled ginger.

Quinoa originated in the Andean region of South America, where it has been a highly valued food for thousands of years. It is usually identified as a grain, but actually it is the seed of the *Chenopodium quinoa* plant, and is related to beets and chard. Quinoa is a great source of magnesium, which is beneficial for blood pressure, heart health, and energy production. It is remarkable for its high amount of protein, which is unusually complete for a plant source in that it includes all nine essential amino acids. Quinoa is a good food to eat for balancing blood sugar; where other refined, low-protein grains contain high amounts of starch that can upset the blood sugar balance, quinoa helps keep blood sugar levels steady.

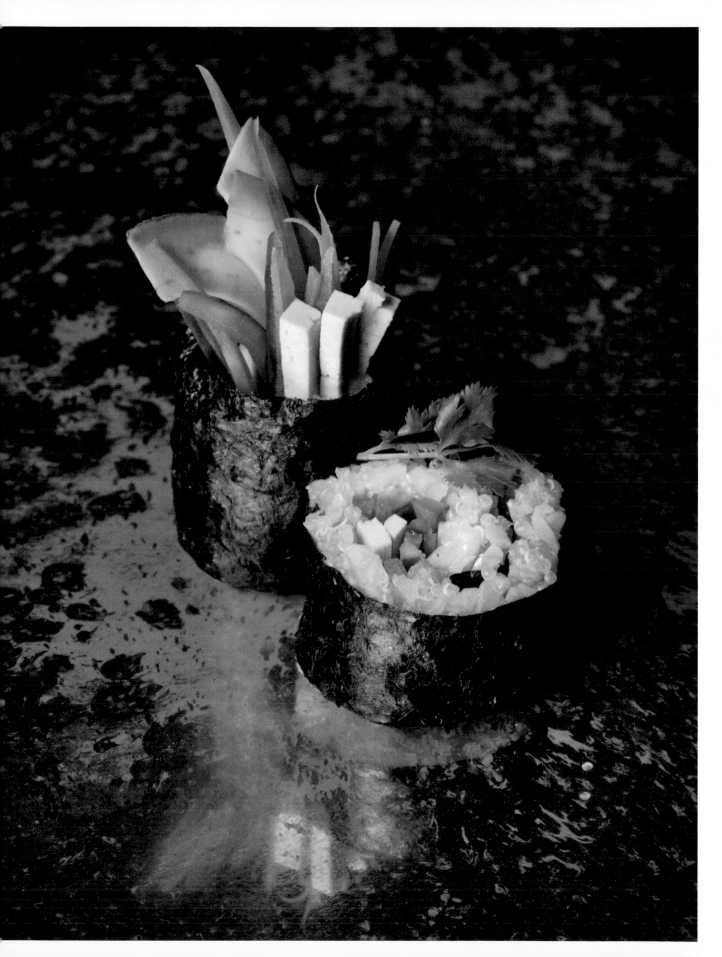

CREAMY CABBAGE

BENEFITS: IMMUNITY + METABOLISM

Another favorite coming from my mother, this recipe is very suitable for vegetarians and those who are lactose-intolerant, but want to enjoy a creamy dish without the dairy. Cabbage comes from the cruciferous family of vegetables; when coupled with shiitake or Chinese mushrooms and soy, these ingredients form a powerful anti-cancer trio that is both easy to prepare and delicious!

SERVES 4

GARNISH

1   handful hijiki seaweed
1   teaspoon grapeseed oil
1   teaspoon soy sauce

1   napa cabbage, cut into 3-inch pieces
½   pound firm tofu, cut into bite-size cubes
1   cup soy milk or coconut milk
2   teaspoons cornstarch
2   tablespoons water
⅓   cup peas, fresh or frozen
2   teaspoons Immunity Spice Blend, pg. 48 (oregano, cilantro, garlic powder, onion powder, star anise, basil, and thyme)
3   dried Chinese mushrooms, soaked in warm water and sliced
2   small tomatoes, chopped
1   stalk celery, finely chopped
¼   red bell pepper, finely chopped
3   cilantro sprigs, chopped
2   teaspoons grapeseed oil

1. Put the hijiki in a bowl, cover with warm water, and soak for 15 minutes. Bring a small saucepan of water to a boil and drop the soaked seaweed into it. Cook for 1 minute, drain, and press on the seaweed to remove excess water. Put the hijiki in a small bowl, stir in the oil and soy sauce, and set aside.

2. Put ½ cup water into a saucepan and bring to a boil over medium-high heat. Add the cabbage, reduce the heat to low, cover, and cook for 15 to 20 minutes, or until the cabbage is soft. Add the tofu, cover, and cook for 3 minutes. Add the soy milk, increase the heat to medium-high, and bring the liquid to a boil.

3. In a small bowl, stir the cornstarch with 2 tablespoons water until dissolved. Slowly pour the mixture into the simmering liquid. Stir until thickened and creamy. Stir in the peas and Immunity Spice Blend and cook for 2 minutes. Transfer the mixture to a wide, deep serving dish and cover to keep warm.

4. Pour about ½ cup water into a skillet and bring to a simmer over medium heat. Add the mushrooms and cook 3 to 4 minutes, until soft. Increase the heat to high, add the tomatoes and celery, and cook for 2 minutes. Pour the mixture over the center of the creamed cabbage.

5. Scatter the hijiki garnish around the dish. Sprinkle the red pepper and cilantro over the cabbage and vegetables, drizzle the oil over the dish, and serve.

Napa cabbage is a popular vegetable in Chinese cuisine, where its sweet, crunchy leaves are much appreciated. Cabbage is a member of the crucifer family of vegetables and is related to broccoli and Brussels sprouts. Like other crucifers, cabbage has amazing anti-cancerous properties, due to its rich source of phytonutrients. Incredibly low in calories and high in fiber, napa cabbage can help aid in weight loss and lower cholesterol. It also offers high levels of vitamin C, vitamin K, and folates, among other important vitamins and minerals that keep you in tip-top shape!

While the **tomato** doesn't play a large role in this recipe, it is still a beneficial fruit worthy of mention! The tomato is notable for its high levels of the antioxidant lycopene, which has been found to reduce the risks of heart disease, macular degeneration, as well as prostate and other cancers. Keep in mind, the lycopene is more available to the body when cooked. Tomatoes are also chock-full of the antioxidant vitamin C and high concentrations of beta-carotene.

MINT PEA FALAFEL

BENEFITS: HEART + ANTI-INFLAMMATION + METABOLISM + DIGESTION

A patient of mine from Iran, whose family fled to the U.S. right before the revolution, attributes his family's longevity to this recipe. Indeed, his grandparents lived to be 98 and 101 eating this family favorite. No wonder! It is a powerhouse grouping of ingredients, from the protein-rich and fat-free peas and garbanzo beans to the heart-healthy garlic and turmeric, to the stomach-settling mint and clove. You can dip the falafel in coconut yogurt or mango chutney—whatever suits your fancy.

SERVES 4

2   cups frozen peas
1   pound dried garbanzo beans, soaked in water overnight
2   large eggs
2   tablespoons avocado oil
1   clove garlic, crushed
1   red chili, seeded and minced
2   scallions, minced
2   tablespoons fresh mint leaves, chopped
1   teaspoon ground turmeric
    Salt and freshly ground black pepper
    Seeds of 1 pomegranate, for garnish
    Plain sheep's milk yogurt, for dipping

1. Preheat the oven to 375°F.

2. Bring a saucepan of water to a boil and add the frozen peas; cook for 1 minute, drain, and rinse under cold running water. Drain the garbanzo beans and transfer them to a food processor. Add the peas, eggs, avocado oil, garlic, chili, scallions, mint, and turmeric and season the mixture with salt and pepper, to taste. Pulse in the food processor until smooth.

3. Using wet hands, roll the mixture into golf ball-size balls and place them on a baking sheet. Bake until just golden, 10 to 12 minutes. Transfer the falafel to a serving platter, garnish with pomegranate seeds on the side of the dish, and serve with yogurt dip.

The garden **pea** we are familiar with today is thought to have originated from a field pea native to central Asia and Europe that has been consumed by humans for thousands of years. Peas have recently been found to be extremely good for the bones. Their content of vitamin K helps maintain high levels of calcium in the bones, while vitamin B_6 and folic acid contribute to healthy collagen and bone matrix formation. Since peas are high in vitamin C, they help boost the immune system, ensure cardiovascular health, and fight cancer.

IMPERIAL CHICKEN INFUSED WITH EIGHT PRECIOUS HERBS

BENEFITS: METABOLISM + ANTI-AGING BEAUTY + SEXUAL HEALTH

If possessing an ageless face with no wrinkles is your dream, look no further than this recipe, which is popularly known among most women in China. Originating from the Imperial Palace, it is considered essential for fertility, longevity, and postpartum rejuvenation. The Eight Precious Herbs formula is traditionally used to fortify energy and build blood—and when combined with chicken, the therapeutic properties are amplified.

SERVES 4

EIGHT PRECIOUS HERBS FORMULA

6	grams angelica root (dang gui)
6	grams white peony (shao yao)
9	grams rehmannia (shou di)
6	grams ligustici (chuang xiong)
6	grams ginseng (ren sheng)
6	grams atractylodis (bai zhu)
6	grams poria (fu ling)
6	grams licorice (gan cao)

1	(3-to-4 pound) whole chicken, rinsed
2	teaspoons salt
8 to 10	dried red jujube dates (hong zao), pitted
5	large slices of fresh ginger (sheng jiang)
2	leeks, sliced
1	small bunch of chives, for garnish

1. Put the 8 precious herbs into a muslin pouch and tie shut.

2. Remove the skin from the chicken and discard. Put the chicken in a stockpot with the herb pouch, salt, dates, ginger, and leeks and fill with enough water to cover the chicken. Bring to a boil over medium-high heat; reduce the heat to medium-low and simmer the chicken until the meat is falling from the bones, about 1 hour.

3. Carefully remove the chicken from the broth and transfer to a plate. Remove and discard the herb pouch. When cool enough to handle, remove the chicken meat from the bones.

4. Serve the chicken meat in small bowls with a scoop of the soup, being sure to ladle some ginger and dates into each bowl. Sprinkle chives over the soup and serve immediately.

The Eight Precious Herbs Formula includes some extremely powerful herbs from the traditional Chinese medical arsenal. You may already be familiar with ginseng as a powerful energy tonic, but you may not know that it also benefits your heart health. Throughout China and Asia, angelica root, or dang gui, has been maintaining women's health for thousands of years, and it has also been found to increase immune function and reduces levels of damaging free radicals in the bloodstream. Licorice helps all the other herbs in this mixture harmonize and become easier to digest. All together, these eight herbs work together to support your supply of vital energy.

SEARED SALMON WITH PICKLED JICAMA

BENEFITS: IMMUNITY + ANTI-INFLAMMATION + METABOLISM

I remember eating this at the home of a couple whose family had come from the Philippines. The Spanish had brought jicama from the New World to the Philippines in the 17th century, and it was embraced in the Philippine cuisine, where it is still often paired with chili or other spices and fish. This was a popular dish in their family back home, and they could boast of healthy grandparents in their eighties and nineties.

SERVES 4

PICKLED JICAMA

1 jicama, peeled and cut into long, thin strips

½ cup apple cider vinegar

SALMON

4 (8-ounce) boneless, skinless salmon fillets

2 tablespoons paprika

1 tablespoon fresh minced garlic

2 teaspoons ground ginger

2 teaspoons ground coriander

2 teaspoons ground cumin

1 teaspoon red chili flakes

2 teaspoons sea salt (or red yeast salt)

Sunflower oil

2 tablespoons chopped fresh cilantro, for garnish

1. To make the pickled jicama, put the jicama in a shallow dish and cover with the vinegar. Refrigerate for 1 hour. Drain well before using.

2. To make the salmon, put the fish on a plate. In a small bowl, mix the paprika, garlic, ginger, coriander, cumin, chili flakes, and salt together until combined. Rub the salmon fillets on all sides with the spice rub; cover and refrigerate for 30 minutes.

3. Cover the bottom of a large nonstick skillet with a very thin layer of sunflower oil and heat over high heat. Sear the salmon for 1 to 2 minutes on each side, depending on thickness. The center should still be rare.

4. Transfer the salmon to serving plates, pile some pickled jicama on top, and garnish with cilantro.

Jicama, sometimes called the Mexican yam, is a white, crisp, and refreshing tuber that has long been a dietary staple in Mexico, Central America, and South America. High in fiber, low in fat, with a very high water content, jicama is an ideal food for weight loss and diabetes management. Jicama also has a high content of vitamin C, which supports the immune system, protects against cancers, and defends against inflammation in the body.

BAKED SALMON WITH LEMON AND MANGO SALSA

BENEFITS: HEART + IMMUNITY + ANTI-INFLAMMATION + DIGESTION + BRAIN & VISION + ANTI-AGING BEAUTY

A friend from Lima, Peru shared this recipe with me. It originally called for tuna, but given the high mercury levels in tuna, I adapted it for salmon. There's a lot to gain from salmon's rich, heart-healthy omega fatty acids. My Peruvian friend remembered his grandmother who lived with his family making this simple dish every Sunday for family brunch. The mango not only adds an exotic tropical flavor, it also contains digestion-assisting enzymes and cancer-preventing phenols. These are good tastes that are good for you! The salsa is great to serve over fish or chicken, and will last for up to 3 days in the refrigerator.

SERVES 4

MANGO SALSA

1 cup diced mango
⅓ cup diced, peeled cucumbers
⅓ cup diced red bell pepper
2 tablespoons chopped fresh mint
2 teaspoons freshly squeezed lime juice

SALMON

½ lemon
1 (1¼-pound) skin-on salmon fillet, rinsed and patted dry
1 cup mango salsa

1. Combine the mango, cucumbers, bell pepper, mint, and lime juice in a bowl and chill.

2. Preheat the oven to 475°F and position a rack in the center of the oven. Line a baking pan with parchment paper.

3. Squeeze the lemon juice onto the parchment paper. Cut the salmon into 4 equal pieces. Set the salmon, skin side down, on the paper-lined pan and spread the salsa evenly over the tops of the fillets. Bake for 10 to 12 minutes, or until the salmon is cooked through. Serve warm.

The omega-3 fatty acids in **salmon** help protect blood vessels from plaque, reduce inflammation, and prevent high blood pressure. Additionally, the combination of niacin and omega-3s in fish protect your brain from Alzheimer's disease and age-related cognitive decline. The omega-3s also lock moisture into skin cells, which contribute to a youthful complexion. Salmon, especially wild-caught salmon, has been found to have lower levels of mercury than many other kinds of fish. This is an all-around great longevity food!

STUFFED SARDINES WITH PESTO

BENEFITS: HEART + ANTI-INFLAMMATION + BRAIN & VISION

One evening I was invited to dinner with an acquaintance from Sicily who had several centenarians in his family. He made this incredible dish for us with sardines that tasted nothing like the ones from cans that I used to consume as a child. Sardines happen to be the cleanest and the healthiest seafood available; they contain the lowest amount of mercury and the highest content of omega-3 fatty acids. This dish is a powerful inflammation fighter—and contains plenty of other benefits for your longevity.

SERVES 4

STUFFING

1 tablespoon grapeseed oil
1 cup coarse corn grits (cornmeal)
2 tablespoons dried cranberries, soaked in water and chopped

SARDINES

12 medium fresh whole sardines
2 tablespoons olive oil
1 teaspoon Heart Spice Blend, pg. 48 (cinnamon, fennel, clove, star anise, white pepper, parsley, ginger, cayenne, and turmeric)
 Salt and freshly ground pepper
 Fresh mint leaves, for garnish

PESTO

 Small handful (about 1 ounce) fresh basil leaves
 Small handful (about 1 ounce) fresh flat-leaf parsley leaves
1 clove garlic, crushed
¼ cup pine nuts, lightly toasted
⅓ cup olive oil
1 lemon, cut into wedges, for garnish

1. Preheat oven to 400°F.

2. To make the stuffing, heat the grapeseed oil in a skillet over medium heat. Stir in the grits and cook, stirring, until golden brown. Stir in the cranberries, remove from the heat, and cool to room temperature.

3. To prepare the sardines, slit each sardine along the belly with a sharp knife and carefully remove the spine; wash and pat the sardines dry. Fill the sardine cavities with the stuffing and transfer them to a baking sheet. Drizzle olive oil over the sardines and sprinkle some herb seasoning over each one. Bake until the fish is cooked through, 10 to 12 minutes. Add the Heart Spice Blend 1 minute before removing from the oven. Remove from the oven and let stand about 5 minutes before serving.

4. Meanwhile, to make the pesto, put the basil, parsley, garlic, pine nuts, and olive oil into a blender or food processor and puree until smooth.

5. Transfer the sardines to a serving dish and drizzle the pesto over them. Garnish with lemon wedges.

With their high levels of omega-3 fatty acids, **sardines** protect your heart and brain health. They are also high in phosphorus, calcium, and potassium, all of which help support your bone health and regulate blood pressure. Small fish like sardines tend to have lower levels of mercury, so they are a smart choice for your health.

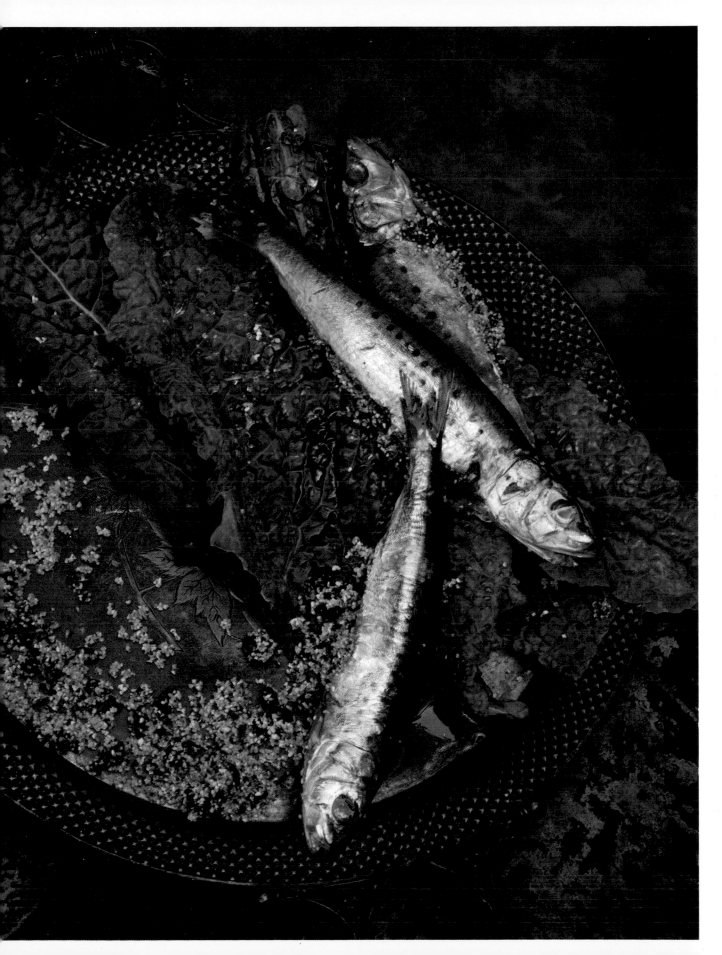

ZESTY HALIBUT IN SOY-GINGER DRESSING

BENEFITS: HEART + IMMUNITY + BRAIN & VISION + ANTI-AGING BEAUTY

Here you've got a tasty recipe that is low-fat, heart-healthy, and good for your circulation. It comes from a Chinese colleague, whose family owned and operated Chinese seafood restaurants for years. This is what they had the chef prepare for them almost every evening when they sat down for dinner. Besides its wonderful taste, it's also a beautiful dish with the colorful peppers.

SERVES 4

1   (2-pound) skin-on halibut fillet, rinsed and patted dry

1   green bell pepper, seeded and cut lengthwise into long, thin strips

1   red bell pepper, seeded and cut lengthwise into long, thin strips

1   yellow bell pepper, seeded and cut lengthwise into long, thin strips

1   medium onion, thinly sliced

1   tablespoon grated fresh ginger

2   teaspoons soy sauce

¼   cup freshly squeezed orange juice

1   tablespoon finely grated orange zest

2   scallions (dark green part only), chopped, for garnish

1. Preheat the oven to 425°F.

2. Put the fish in a baking dish and top with the bell peppers, onion, ginger, and soy sauce. Drizzle the orange juice over the fish and sprinkle the zest evenly over it; cover the dish tightly with parchment paper. Bake for 15 minutes, or until the fish is cooked through.

3. Using two large spatulas, transfer the fish to a serving platter, pour the juices from the baking dish over the top, and garnish with the scallions.

Tangy and crunchy, **bell peppers** come in a rainbow of colors. They are packed with vitamins C and A, two antioxidants that work together to neutralize free radicals. Their content of beta-carotene, the vitamin A precursor, supports vision health and skin regeneration. Among many beneficial vitamins, peppers contain vitamin B_6, folic acid, and fiber—all helpful for protection against hardening of the arteries and heart disease. Compared with green peppers, red peppers contain more vitamins and nutrients, especially lycopene, a carotenoid that can help protect against certain cancers such as prostate and cervical cancers.

BLACK BASS WITH CORIANDER

BENEFITS: HEART + ANTI-INFLAMMATION + DIGESTION + ANTI-AGING BEAUTY

Originally created for the emperors and empresses of China to support their health and longevity pursuits, this dish was very popular with Emperor Qianlong of the Qing Dynasty who lived to 89 years of age—a rarity in the 1700s and among Chinese royals. Secret ingredients make this bass dish a special treat! Coriander and other spices will boost your circulation and lower your cholesterol, as well as make your hair, nails, tendons, and ligaments strong and flexible.

SERVES 6

CORIANDER SPICE MIX
½ teaspoon ground coriander
½ teaspoon finely ground black pepper
½ teaspoon ground cloves
½ teaspoon ground cinnamon
½ teaspoon ground fennel seed
½ teaspoon ground star anise
½ teaspoon ground turmeric

1 (3-pound) skin-on black bass fillet, washed and patted dry
2 large banana leaves
2 tablespoons chopped fresh cilantro
3 cloves garlic, chopped
1 tablespoon grated fresh ginger
1 teaspoon salt
1 tablespoon light soy sauce
  Cilantro sprigs, for garnish
  Orange wedges, for garnish

1. To make the spice mix, stir all of the spices together in a small bowl.

2. Put the fish in a shallow dish, rub the spice mix evenly over the flesh, and refrigerate for 1 hour.

3. Preheat the oven to 375°F. Lay a large sheet of parchment paper on a work surface, stack the banana leaves, and set them on the paper. Put the bass fillet on the center of the leaves and sprinkle the cilantro, garlic, ginger, and salt over the fish. Drizzle the soy sauce over the fish. Wrap the fish tightly in the banana leaves, then wrap the packet tightly in the paper. Transfer to a baking dish and bake for 25 minutes.

4. Unwrap the fish, discard the paper, and set the packet on a serving platter. Open the banana leaves, exposing the fish, and garnish with cilantro sprigs and orange wedges. Serve immediately.

This **coriander spice mix** packs a punch of flavor and healthy benefits! Coriander seeds have possible anti-diabetic, anti-inflammatory, and cholesterol-lowering properties, and peppercorns promote intestinal health. Cinnamon has been linked to lowered blood sugar, helpful for improving insulin sensitivity and lowering cholesterol. Cloves and star anise improve digestive function, while fennel seeds boost production of gastric juices and soothe the nervous system. Turmeric boasts anti-inflammatory, antioxidant, and anti-tumor properties. If you are on medication, speak with your physician to make sure these spices aren't interfering with your medicine.

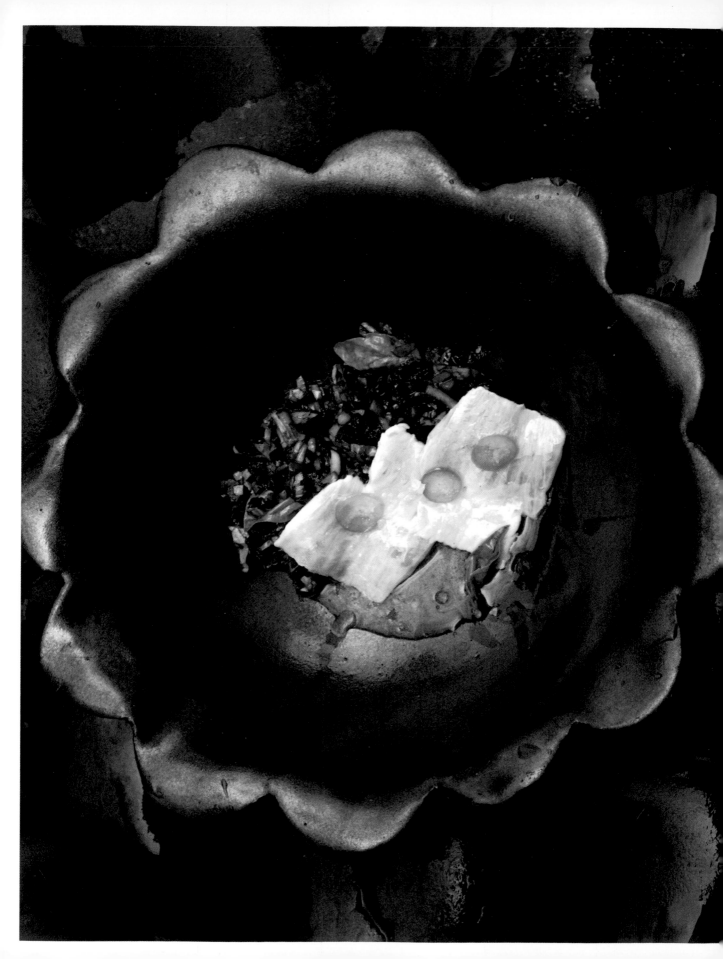

HALIBUT CRUDO

BENEFITS: HEART + BRAIN & VISION

Crudo means "raw" in Italian, and in the fishing villages of Italy, thin slices of raw fish are often served with whatever is on hand—such as olive oil, lemon, and basil. This delicacy was introduced to me a while back by a friend of mine who owns a house in Puglia, a coastal fishing town in southern Italy. The raw fish is marinated and "cooked" by the citric acid of lemon juice. It is then seasoned with herbs and spices that make the fish easily digestible—not to mention delicious. No wonder it has become wildly popular in hip restaurants throughout the U.S.!

SERVES 4

1½ pounds very fresh, sushi-grade skinless, boneless halibut fillet

2 tablespoons freshly squeezed lemon juice

1 tablespoon freshly squeezed ginger juice

1 teaspoon sea salt

¼ cup extra-virgin olive oil

3 red radishes, thinly sliced

6 black olives, pitted and chopped

8 fresh basil leaves, chopped

1 small jalapeño pepper, sliced paper-thin

1. Cut the halibut fillet into very thin slices and transfer the slices to a shallow dish. Season the fish with salt and drizzle the lemon, ginger juice, and 3 tablespoons of the olive oil over the top. Cover the dish with plastic wrap and let it marinate in the refrigerator for 30 minutes.

2. Meanwhile, mix the radishes, olives, basil, and remaining olive oil together in a small bowl. To serve, divide the radish mixture among 4 salad plates and arrange it on one half of each plate. Arrange one-quarter of the halibut slices on the empty side of each plate, drizzle some of the marinade over the fish, and garnish each plate with the jalapeño slices.

While the omega-rich **halibut** is the star of this recipe, basil plays an important supporting role in the flavor and healing benefits. Basil is filled with luteolin, a bioflavonoid that is considered one of the best protective substances of cell DNA from radiation. These potent antioxidants help combat the effects of aging and protect against cancer. Basil is a great herb to grow in a sunny kitchen window during the bright summer months, so you can have easy access to its tasty leaves while cooking.

MISO-GLAZED SOLE WITH SWISS CHARD

BENEFITS: HEART + IMMUNITY + ANTI-INFLAMMATION

This is absolutely one of my favorite dishes! The soft, flavorful fish is placed on top of tender, but textured, chard leaves, a combination that is similar to chicken in lettuce cups—but this version is much juicier. Swiss chard is considered one of the most nutritious vegetables, possessing flavonoids that regulate blood sugar along with antioxidant and anti-inflammatory properties. It also helps build strong bones with vitamin K.

SERVES 4

MARINADE

3   tablespoons low-sodium white miso
3   tablespoons sake or white wine
2   tablespoons honey
2   tablespoons soy sauce

1½ pound piece boneless, skinless sole fillet, cut into four 4-inch pieces
1   bunch Swiss chard, woody stems removed
2   tablespoons grapeseed oil
2   teaspoons black sesame seeds

1. To make the marinade, put the miso, sake, honey, and soy sauce in a saucepan and slowly warm it over low heat, stirring occasionally, until smooth. Remove from the heat and let it cool.

2. Put the sole fillets in a shallow glass dish and pour the marinade over, cover with plastic wrap, and refrigerate overnight.

3. Bring ¼ cup water to a boil in a skillet over medium-high heat, add the Swiss chard, and cook until just tender, 4 to 5 minutes, taking care not to tear the leaves. Remove from the heat, pat the leaves dry, and spread them out evenly on 4 serving plates.

4. Heat the oil in the same skillet over high heat and place the fish in the pan, then sprinkle the sesame seeds over. Cook fish for 1 minute on each side. Pour the marinade into the pan, reduce the heat to low, and simmer for 2 minutes. Remove the fish carefully, taking care not to break apart the fillets, and arrange 1 piece on top of the chard leaves on each plate.

5. Drizzle the remaining pan sauce evenly over the fish and serve immediately.

Miso is a traditional Japanese seasoning that is usually made from fermented soybeans. Like other legume-based foods, soy miso is a good source of fiber and protein. Miso also contains a wide variety of phytonutrients, which can function as antioxidants and anti-inflammatory substances. Soy miso is being investigated for its possible cardiovascular, anti-cancer, and digestive benefits, and it is speculated that these benefits are due to the antioxidants in miso that result from the fermentation process. Due to the widespread use of GMOs in U.S. soybean production, look for certified organic soy miso, and for your health, choose low-sodium.

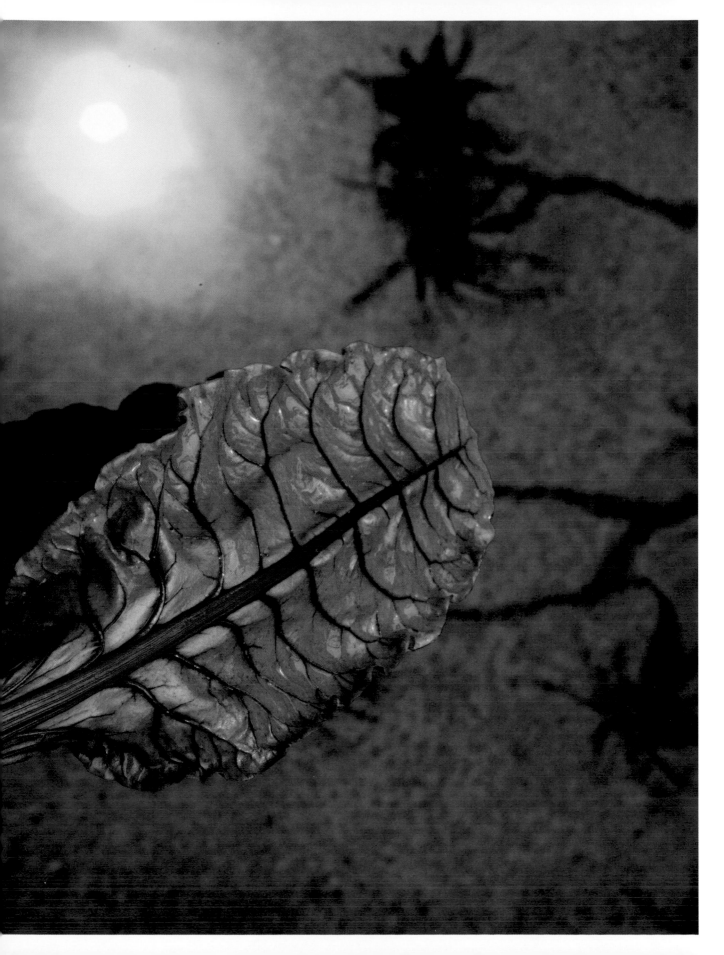

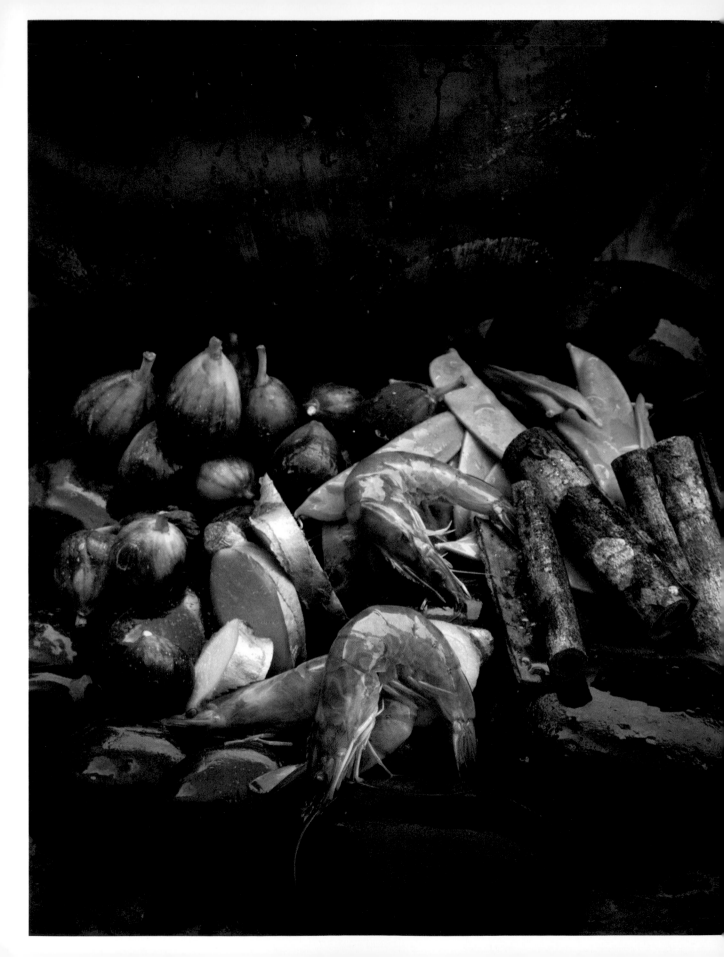

SAUTÉED KING PRAWNS WITH CHESTNUTS AND FIGS

BENEFITS: HEART + METABOLISM + DIGESTION + SEXUAL HEALTH

This recipe came from the imperial palace of China and was designed to boost the sexual vitality of the emperors. Chinese medicine has long considered prawns, chestnuts, and figs to be tonics for the kidney/adrenal systems, which are considered fundamental to the health of the sexual systems. Figs are thought to increase sperm production and motility, and chestnuts are rich in folate and zinc, important for the production of sex hormones. Prawns are rich in B vitamins, zinc, and heart-healthy omega-3 fatty acids. What's good for your heart is good for your sex, too!

SERVES 4

20 dried, peeled chestnuts, soaked in hot water for 1 hour
12 ounces king prawns, shelled and deveined
1 teaspoon salt
1 teaspoon white pepper
3 fresh black figs (or dried figs soaked in warm water to reconstitute)
⅓ cup port
3 tablespoons rice bran oil
½ cup snow peas
1 scallion, sliced into long, thin pieces
4 slices fresh ginger, peeled and sliced into matchsticks
1 tablespoon dark soy sauce
1 cinnamon stick
3 whole star anise

1. Bring a saucepan of water to a boil and cook the chestnuts until slightly soft, about 30 minutes; drain and let stand until cool.

2. Rub the shrimp with salt and white pepper. Quarter the figs lengthwise, put them into a small bowl, and pour the port over them. Let stand for 10 minutes; drain and reserve the port.

3. Preheat a wok over high heat for 2 to 3 minutes, then add the vegetable oil and heat until rippling. Carefully add the shrimp and stir-fry briefly; remove them from the wok as soon as the color changes and transfer them to a plate.

4. Add the snow peas, drained figs, scallion, and ginger to the wok and stir-fry for 2 to 3 minutes. Transfer to the plate with the shrimp.

5. Add the chestnuts, reserved port, soy sauce, cinnamon stick, and star anise to the wok and simmer until the sauce is reduced and thickened. Return the cooked shrimp and vegetables to the wok and simmer, stirring occasionally, for another 2 to 3 minutes. Remove the cinnamon stick and star anise, transfer to a large shallow bowl, and serve immediately.

Figs have long had a reputation in traditional medicine of being a natural laxative. Indeed, they have a good content of fiber, potassium, magnesium, and calcium—all helpful for cardiovascular health. The high fiber content may also help with weight management. The calcium content is fairly high for a fruit and will support your bone health. If you are sensitive to sulfites, seek out a sulfite-free version of figs.

LEMON CHICKEN WITH ARTICHOKE HEARTS

BENEFITS: IMMUNITY + DIGESTION

This recipe was shared with me by a friend from Israel and prominently features artichokes, which are very high in potent antioxidants that support liver and gall bladder function while helping to prevent cancer. This simple and tasty chicken dish is quick to prepare and great for your health.

SERVES 4

½ cup rice flour
1 teaspoon salt
¼ teaspoon freshly ground pepper
4 boneless, skinless chicken breasts
¼ cup extra virgin olive oil
2 cups chicken broth
   Juice of 1 lemon
1 (10-ounce) jar marinated artichoke hearts, drained and coarsely chopped
2 tablespoons fresh minced sage leaves
   Cooked Brown Rice with Pine Nuts, pg. 125, for serving
   Fresh vegetables, for serving

1. Combine the flour, salt, and pepper in a resealable plastic storage bag. Place 1 chicken breast at a time in the flour mixture, seal the bag, and shake to coat; transfer to a plate. Repeat with the remaining chicken.

2. Heat the oil in a large nonstick skillet over medium heat. Add the chicken and cook, turning once, until browned and cooked through, about 8 minutes total. Transfer the chicken to a warmed platter and cover to keep warm.

3. Add the broth and lemon juice to the same skillet; bring to a boil. Boil until the liquid is reduced to about 1 cup. Stir in the chopped artichokes and simmer until very hot.

4. Transfer the chicken to 4 serving plates and pour the sauce over. Serve with brown rice sprinkled with pine nuts and fresh vegetables.

A native of the Mediterranean, the **artichoke** belongs to the thistle tribe of the sunflower family. The artichoke "vegetable" that we eat is actually the plant's flower bud. Artichoke is considered a potent liver protector due to its content of a flavonoid called silymarin, which has potent antioxidant properties. Nutritionally, the artichoke is a good source of vitamin C, folate, and potassium. This diuretic vegetable also helps improve digestion and reduce cholesterol levels.

MARMALADE CHICKEN BROCHETTES

BENEFITS: HEART + IMMUNITY + METABOLISM + DIGESTION

My Persian friends from Iran, who are proud of their long-lived ancestors, shared this recipe with me. The spices cardamom, cinnamon, and ginger are full of volatile oils that aid digestion, boost fertility and balance blood sugar—to name just a few of their benefits! Citrus peel contains high levels of vitamin C and also PMFs, or polymethoxylated flavones, which have been found to prevent diabetes and lower cholesterol. With all its amazing beneficial properties, this incredibly tasty dish should be experienced by all!

SERVES 4

MARINADE

3	tablespoons lemon marmalade or preserves
1	clove garlic, crushed
1	1-inch piece fresh ginger, peeled and grated
½	teaspoon ground cinnamon
½	teaspoon ground cardamom
3	tablespoons olive oil
1½	pounds boneless, skinless chicken thighs, cut into 1-inch cubes
3	tablespoons grapeseed oil
10 to 12	large pitted green olives
1	cucumber, peeled, seeded, and cut into ¾-inch cubes
2	tablespoons minced chives
1	teaspoon red chili flakes
	Wooden skewers, about 6 inches

1. To make the marinade, whisk the marmalade, garlic, ginger, cinnamon, cardamom, and olive oil in a large bowl until combined. Toss the chicken pieces in the marinade until coated, cover, and refrigerate overnight.

2. Heat the oil in a nonstick skillet over medium-high heat and cook the chicken pieces for 1 to 2 minutes on each side, or until cooked through. Transfer the chicken to a plate and cover to keep warm. While the pan is still hot, add the olives and cucumber and stir-fry briefly. Transfer the vegetables to the plate with the chicken.

3. Thread one cucumber cube, one piece of chicken, and one olive onto each wooden skewer, in that order, and repeat to fill up the skewer. Transfer the brochettes to a serving dish and sprinkle the chives and chili flakes over them to garnish. Serve immediately.

Traditionally, **lemon peel** has been used to aid digestion by helping to reduce gas and cramping in the digestive system. Citrus peels may contribute to lower risks of heart disease by virtue of their polymethoxylated flavone (PMF) compounds. These PMFs and the limonene content of citrus are thought to balance blood sugar, activate liver detoxification, and lower cholesterol. Citrus peels also contain high levels of antioxidants, which, when combined with the high vitamin C content of citrus peel, may help protect your DNA from cancer-causing damage. Who knew marmalade had so much to offer?

HONEY-GLAZED MASALA CHICKEN WITH APRICOTS

BENEFITS: DIGESTION

One of the staple foods of the famously long-living centenarians in the Hunza Valley of the Himalayas is the apricot. Masala chicken is a popular Indian dish. People not used to the spiciness of masala may find it a little strong, but adding the apricots gives it a mild sweet-and-sour taste, balancing the spiciness of the masala.

SERVES 4

2   tablespoons olive oil
2   medium onions, sliced
2   cloves garlic, finely chopped
1   1-inch piece fresh ginger,
     peeled and finely chopped
1½ teaspoons masala spice (ground
     cumin, ground cinnamon,
     ground clove, bay leaf, ground
     peppercorn, ground coriander,
     ground cardamom)
3   pounds boneless, skinless
     chicken pieces (thigh and
     breast), cut into 2-inch chunks
2   tablespoons tomato puree
1   teaspoon fine sea salt
1   cup water
2   tablespoons rice vinegar
10   dried apricots
2   tablespoons honey
     Chopped fresh parsley, for garnish

1. Heat the oil in a deep skillet over medium heat. Add the onions and cook, stirring occasionally, until softened. Stir in the garlic, ginger, and masala. Add the chicken pieces and stir-fry until cooked through, about 5 minutes.

2. Add the tomato puree, salt, and 1 cup water; bring to a boil. Reduce the heat to low, cover, and simmer for 20 minutes.

3. Uncover the skillet, add the vinegar and apricots, stir well, cover, and simmer 15 minutes more. Transfer the chicken to a serving platter, drizzle honey over the top, and garnish with parsley.

Masala can spice up your circulation! Many of the everyday cooking seasonings in our spice rack are actually spices and herbs that possess powerful healing properties. For example, cinnamon and coriander have been clinically shown to prevent blood clots and improve circulation. One of my favorite spice mixes is the Indian blend masala. It is not "tongue-burning" but rather a gentle, tummy-warming spice mix that improves digestion, absorption, and helps reduce abdominal bloat.

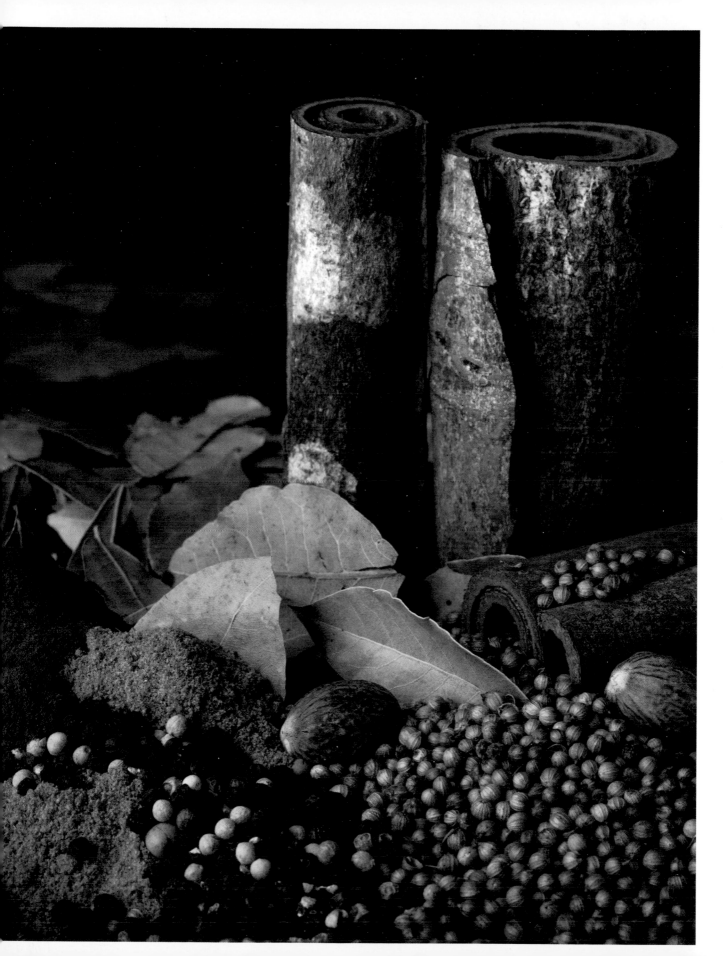

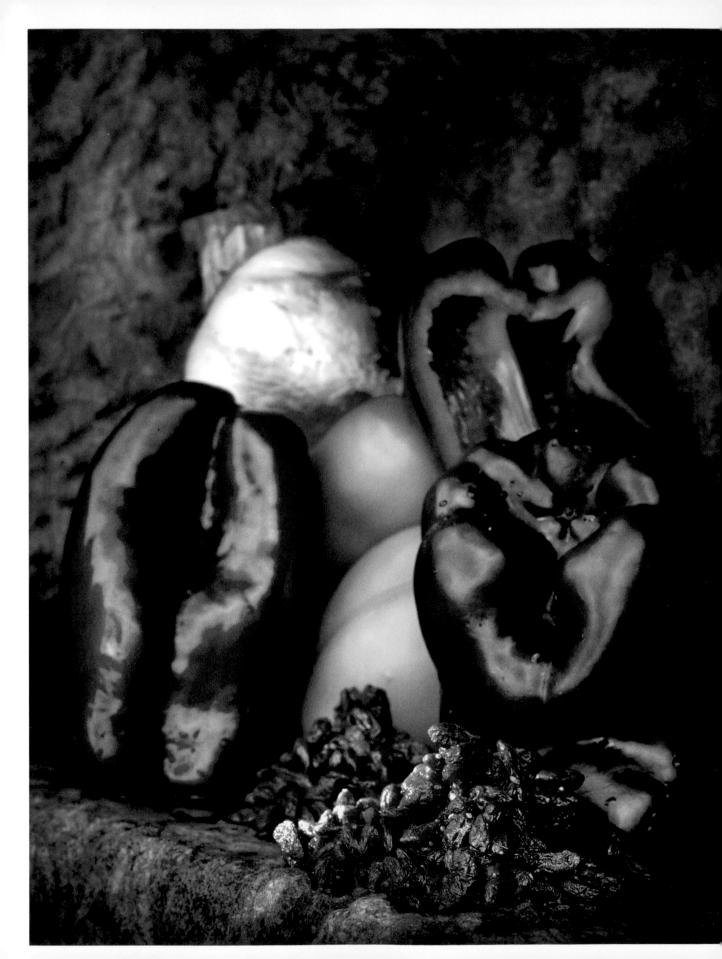

SPICY TRI-COLOR PEPPER BEEF WITH HIMALAYAN GOJI BERRIES

BENEFITS: IMMUNITY + METABOLISM + BRAIN & VISION

Goji berries are the tasty orange-colored berries that grow in the Himalayan mountain range. They are rich in antioxidant carotenoids and vitamin C, and are used in Chinese medicine for boosting brain function, strengthening vision, and bolstering immunity. This recipe is popular among centenarians in the northern part of China, where beef is more readily available.

SERVES 4

SAUCE

1 tablespoon light soy sauce
1 tablespoon chili bean sauce
1 tablespoon sherry
1 teaspoon rice vinegar
½ teaspoon sugar

STIR-FRY

3 tablespoons rice bran oil
1 pound beef tenderloin fillet, sliced into thin strips
1 sweet onion, chopped
1 green bell pepper, cored, seeded, and thinly sliced lengthwise
1 yellow bell pepper, cored, seeded, and thinly sliced lengthwise
1 scallion, sliced crosswise into ½-inch pieces
¼ cup dried goji berries, soaked in warm water for 15 minutes and drained
1 teaspoon salt
½ teaspoon freshly ground black pepper

1. To make the sauce, whisk the soy sauce, chili sauce, sherry, vinegar, and sugar together in a small bowl until dissolved. Set aside.

2. To make the stir-fry, heat a wok over high heat for 2 to 3 minutes until very hot. Add the oil, and when rippling, add the sliced beef, onion, and bell peppers to the wok and stir-fry for about 4 to 5 minutes, until the onions begin to soften and the meat is beginning to brown. Pour the sauce over the beef, add the scallion, drained goji berries, salt, and pepper, and toss well to mix. Let the sauce bubble for 2 to 3 minutes until the juice thickens.

3. Transfer to a warm serving dish and serve immediately.

Goji berries have been used in traditional Chinese medicine for thousands of years for their tonic effects on vision and the brain. They are remarkable for having one of the highest concentrations of antioxidant carotenoids, especially beta-carotene, of just about any plant in the world—that's a major health accomplishment! In addition to their high antioxidant activity, these superfood berries have anti-inflammatory properties. They are eaten to enhance immunity, improve eyesight, protect the liver, improve circulation, boost sperm count, lower cholesterol, and restore energy. Goji berries are easy to find now in almost all health-food stores.

SNACKS

The flavorful snack recipes here will help you round out your five small meals a day and are easy to bring with you wherever you go. A healthy snack at mid-morning and another at mid-afternoon can keep your energy running smoothly, bring you a burst of nutrients, and cut back on the kind of cravings that lead to a fast food frenzy at your next break.

These savory snacks include everything you would want out of a calorie-packed bag of chips: they feature big, tasty flavors with an element of pleasing crisp texture. Best of all, you will find plenty of high-quality ingredients that will contribute to your health and longevity for years down the road. Enjoy!

Great Grab-and-Go Snacks
These are excellent snacks, both for their portability and for their healthy attributes.

- apples, with or without nut butter
- oranges
- bananas
- grapes
- berries
- dried fruits
- half an avocado with a squeeze of lime juice and cilantro
- sliced veggies like cucumbers, bell peppers, celery, broccoli, and carrots
- edamame
- nuts and seeds
- seaweed chips
- rice cake chips
- veggie chips
- olives
- yogurt, including soy, coconut, or rice milk
- hard-boiled eggs
- smoothie or juice made from fresh fruit, veggies, and herbs

ANTI-AGING BRAIN MIX

BENEFITS: HEART + IMMUNITY + ANTI-INFLAMMATION + METABOLISM
+ BRAIN & VISION + ANTI-AGING BEAUTY

This snack is a real anti-aging boon to your brain! Packed with protein and essential fatty acids, it is also chock-full of the amino arginine, which stimulates the pituitary gland at the base of the brain to release growth hormone, a substance that declines quickly after age thirty-five. The berries offer their own antioxidant benefits. Feel free to substitute dried cranberries for the goji berries if you prefer.

MAKES 6 SERVINGS

1   cup walnuts
½ cup pine nuts
¼ cup sesame seeds
½ cup pumpkin seeds
⅓ cup dried goji berries
½ cup dried apricots
½ cup dried blueberries

Mix the ingredients together and pack the mix in a sealed container or resealable bag to preserve freshness. Eat a small handful between meals every day as a snack. This mix of nuts and fruits supplies essential fatty acids, carotenoids, and anti-oxidants that will maintain a steady supply of fuel and energy for your brain.

With its two lobes that resemble a brain, **walnuts** aptly advertise their cognitive benefits. Rich in omega-3 essential fatty acids, walnuts protect cardiovascular health, improve cognitive function, and possess anti-inflammatory benefits that are helpful for asthma, rheumatoid arthritis, and inflammatory skin diseases like eczema and psoriasis. Additionally, walnuts contain the antioxidant compound ellagic acid, which supports the immune system and is thought to have many anti-cancer properties.

BLACK BEAN HUMMUS

BENEFITS: HEART + IMMUNITY + METABOLISM + SEXUAL HEALTH

Hummus is widely enjoyed all over the world. The Chinese centenarians I met consume very large amounts of hummus. Chickpeas, while delicious, are just the tip of the hummus iceberg! Hummus can be made out of any bean or legume, including black beans, mung beans, and adzuki beans. Whatever bean you choose, you will be benefiting from a high-fiber, low-fat, high-protein snack. The lignans in beans and legumes are beneficial for the immune system and hormonal health, and helpful for women going through menopause. Some good chip alternatives to pair with this hummus include vegetable sticks, seaweed chips, veggie chips, rice cake chips, or another light, gluten-free food.

SERVES 3

2   cups cooked black beans,
    or 1 16-ounce can
1   clove garlic, minced
    Juice of 1 lemon
2   tablespoons sesame tahini
1   tablespoon olive oil
1   tablespoon honey
1   tablespoon sesame seeds
1   pinch of cayenne pepper
    Salt and freshly ground pepper
1   sprig cilantro, for garnish

Put black beans, garlic, lemon juice, tahini, olive oil, and honey into a food processor or blender and puree until smooth. Toast sesame seeds until slightly golden and add to food processor and puree, along with more olive oil, until desired consistency is achieved. Season with salt and pepper to taste. Serve in dipping dish and garnish with cilantro.

I am a fan of hummus made from any bean, but I especially like it when it is made from **black beans**, which are on my top-ten longevity food list. Like many other legumes, black beans are a very good source of cholesterol-lowering dietary fiber and are beneficial for your cardiovascular health. One cup of black beans will supply almost *three-quarters* of your daily value for dietary fiber. They are also rich in iron, which helps increase your energy level, and they are as rich as cranberries in the antioxidant compounds anthocyanins, which help protect against cancer. When combined with a whole grain, black beans become a complete source of protein, a great boon to vegetarians looking for protein alternatives to meat.

AVOCADO HUMMUS

BENEFITS: HEART + IMMUNITY + ANTI-INFLAMMATION + METABOLISM + CLEANSING
+ BRAIN & VISION + ANTI-AGING BEAUTY + SEXUAL HEALTH

This is a fresh twist on the chickpea hummus found in Middle Eastern cuisine. The chickpeas offer a good content of cholesterol-lowering fiber, and the avocado is not only rich in heart-healthy monounsaturated fat, but it is also an excellent source of the antioxidant glutathione, which helps regulate the immune system. Enjoy!

SERVES 4

2   cups cooked chickpeas,
    or 1 16-ouncecan
1   clove garlic, minced
    Juice of 1 lemon
2   tablespoons sesame tahini
1   tablespoon olive oil
1   tablespoon honey
1   tablespoon sesame seeds
1   avocado, pitted and peeled
1   pinch of cayenne pepper
    Salt and freshly ground pepper
1   teaspoon paprika, for garnish

Put chickpeas, garlic, lemon juice, tahini, olive oil, and honey into a food processor or blender and puree until smooth. Toast sesame seeds until slightly golden and add into puree along with avocado, and puree until creamy. Add more olive oil until desired consistency is achieved, then season with salt and pepper to taste. Serve in dipping dish and garnish with paprika.

Garbanzo beans, or chickpeas, are a good source of cholesterol-lowering fiber. In addition, garbanzos' high fiber content prevents blood sugar levels from rising too rapidly after a meal, making these beans an especially good choice for individuals with diabetes, insulin resistance, or hypoglycemia. Garbanzo beans help you feel full with their fiber content and are frequently recommended for weight loss plans. In traditional Chinese medicine, it is said that garbanzos help with some inflammatory skin conditions, like psoriasis and eczema.

EDAMAME HUMMUS

BENEFITS: HEART + METABOLISM + SEXUAL HEALTH

With this snack, you get heart-healthy benefits from the flaxseeds and the sesame tahini. The essential fatty acids and dietary fiber of the edamame are also beneficial, and they give this hummus a distinctly Asian flavor.

SERVES 4

2 cups cooked soy edamame beans or 1 16-ounce bag frozen, ready to serve edamame

1 clove garlic, minced
Juice of 1 lemon

2 tablespoons sesame tahini

1 tablespoon olive oil

1 tablespoon honey

1 tablespoon flaxseeds

1 pinch of cayenne pepper
Salt and freshly ground pepper

1 sprig cilantro, for garnish

Put edamame beans, garlic, lemon juice, tahini, olive oil, and honey into a food processor or blender and puree until smooth. Toast flaxseeds and add to food processor and puree, along with more olive oil until achieving desired consistency. Season with salt and pepper to taste. Serve in dipping dish and garnish with cilantro.

Low in fat, low in cholesterol, and high in protein, **edamame** boasts a high content of essential fatty acids and dietary fiber, as well as numerous minerals and vitamins, such as folic acid, manganese, and vitamin K. Of course, edamame should be avoided by anyone who is allergic to soy.

SOY YOGURT DIP WITH CARROTS, JICAMA, AND CUCUMBER STICKS

BENEFITS: HEART + DIGESTION + BRAIN & VISION

Soy yogurt is a modern adaptation of a sweet soy dish that has been eaten in China for a long time. It is a great substitute for dairy and pairs well with cut vegetables. Soy yogurt is a low-fat, high-protein snack that provides beneficial bacteria for your gut. Most people don't realize the wonderful benefits that cucumbers have! High in vitamin A, they reduce inflammation and have incredible anti-cancer properties. Carrots are full of fiber and beta-carotene. These are the two I like best, but you can use any veggies that you like.

SERVES 4

2 large carrots, peeled and cut into 3-inch long sticks

2 large cucumbers, peeled and seeded and cut into 3-inch long sticks

1 jicama, peeled and cut into 3-inch long sticks

2 sprigs of parley, for garnish

4 8-ounce containers plain soy yogurt

2 cloves garlic, minced

1 tablespoon fresh basil, minced

1 tablespoon fresh parsley, minced

Arrange carrot, cucumber, and jícama sticks on a serving platter. In a serving bowl, mix yogurt, garlic, parsley, and basil and place on the platter. Garnish with sprigs of parsley.

Carrots are famous for their ability to brighten eyesight. Their characteristic orange color comes from a high content of beta-carotene, which is metabolized into vitamin A, the substance in carrots that helps improve vision, especially night vision. Beta-carotene not only improves eyesight, it can also delay the onset of aging and protect our skin from the sun's damaging rays. Additionally, carrots have a high vitamin C content, a great support for your immune system.

GUACAMOLE WITH KALE CHIPS

BENEFITS: IMMUNITY + BRAIN & VISION

A caterer friend of mine from the Czech Republic in Eastern Europe shared these kale chips with guacamole, and I was so taken with their delicious taste. Kale is such a healthy green vegetable, but I frankly never liked kale until I tried this recipe. Try it out!

SERVES 4

KALE CHIPS

1   bunch kale, woody stems removed, cut into 2-inch pieces
1   tablespoon olive oil
    Salt and freshly ground black pepper

GUACAMOLE

2   ripe Hass avocados
1   stalk celery, finely diced
1   tablespoon dried goji berries, soaked in cold water for 1 hour, drained, and patted dry
½   teaspoon paprika
1   teaspoon pickled ginger, finely chopped
2   scallions, finely chopped
    Juice of 1 lemon

1. To make the chips, preheat the oven to 350°F. Line a baking sheet with parchment paper.

2. Pat the kale pieces dry and spread them evenly in a single layer on the baking sheet. Drizzle the oil over the kale and sprinkle the salt and pepper over the top. Bake for 10 to 15 minutes, until slightly browned and crisp but not burnt. Immediately remove them from the oven and let them cool on the pan.

3. To make the guacamole, cut the avocados in half, remove the pit, and scoop out the flesh into a bowl. Add the celery, goji berries, paprika, ginger, scallions, and lemon juice and mash together until completely mixed.

4. Serve with kale chips.

A member of the crucifer family, **kale** has incredible benefits for your health. Like other cruciferous vegetables, kale is a rich source of the antioxidant phytonutrients that help cleanse the body of cancer-causing substances. Kale leaves provide more nutritional value for fewer calories than almost any other food. Kale is rich in beta-carotene, vitamin K, vitamin C, manganese, and dietary fiber, among many other nutrients. Kale's content of calcium helps build bones, vitamin E may play a role in lowering risk of cognitive decline, and the carotenoids found in kale support vision health. This is one green that is worth loving!

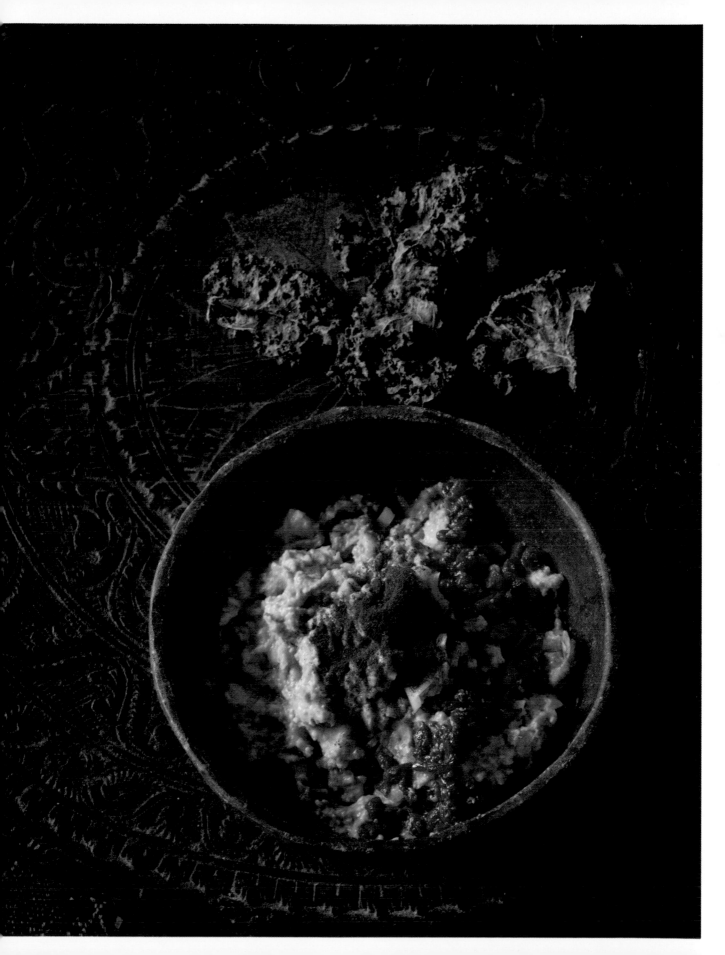

BAKED SWEET POTATO CHIPS WITH PUMPKIN SEEDS

BENEFITS: IMMUNITY + ANTI-INFLAMMATION

I learned about this delicious snack when I was in China, interviewing a 102-year-old former doctor in Sichuan Province. He loved to snack on these chips made from these two powerful longevity foods.

SERVES 4

3 large sweet potatoes, washed and scrubbed, sliced into ⅛-inch thick slices

3 tablespoons pumpkin seeds, lightly crushed in food processor

¼ cup grapeseed oil

¼ teaspoon ground cinnamon

1 tablespoon chives, minced

1 clove garlic, minced

1 teaspoon cayenne pepper

A pinch of salt

Preheat oven to 375°F. Place all ingredients in a mixing bowl and toss to coat sweet potato slices. Lay sweet potato slices on a baking sheet and bake for 20 minutes, turning slices over halfway through. Remove promptly to avoid burning. Let cool and serve by themselves or with Avocado Hummus (page 169).

Crunchy and satisfying, **pumpkin seeds,** sometimes called "pepitas," are much more than just snacks. They are high in zinc, which is a natural protector against bone loss, contain almost your whole daily requirement of magnesium, promote prostate health, reduce inflammation, help lower LDL cholesterol, and prevent kidney stones. These green seeds also contain the powerful antioxidant L-cysteine, which can help protect your body from the harmful effects of pollution, chemicals, radiation, alcohol, and smoke. This naturally occurring amino acid may also help boost the immune system, defend against heart disease, build muscle, and minimize fat buildup.

GLUTEN-FREE OLIVE BREAD

BENEFITS: ANTI-INFLAMMATION

A colleague of mine from Spain, a practicing doctor for more than thirty years, shared this recipe with me. He adapted this bread recipe to accommodate his gluten-sensitive patients. Multiple kinds of flour are used, which gives you a much more diverse nutritional profile than just wheat. Olives have excellent benefits of their own, including antioxidant and anti-inflammatory properties. This is an absolutely delicious bread that would be welcome at any table. The bread can also be made in a bread machine. Just prepare the dough as below and follow the manufacturer's instructions with your machine.

MAKES 1 LOAF

½ cup warm water
1 tablespoon active dry yeast
1 cup brown rice flour
1 cup white rice flour
⅓ cup chickpea flour
⅓ cup potato flour
⅓ cup tapioca flour
1 tablespoon xanthan gum
1 teaspoon sea salt
2 eggs, beaten
¼ cup avocado oil
¼ cup maple syrup
1 teaspoon vinegar
¼ cup chopped pitted black olives

1. Preheat the oven to 375°F. Put the water in a small bowl and sprinkle the yeast over it. Let stand about 10 minutes, until foamy.

2. Meanwhile, in a large bowl, whisk the brown and white rice flours, chickpea flour, potato flour, tapioca flour, xanthan gum, and salt together until combined. In another bowl, whisk the yeast mixture, eggs, oil, syrup, vinegar, and olives together until well combined. Pour the wet ingredients into the dry and mix well with a wooden spoon until a thick dough forms and there are no longer any lumps of flour. Pour the batter into a large loaf pan and bake in the center of the oven until risen, firm, and a tester inserted in the center comes out clean, about 45 minutes.

3. Let the bread cool completely in the pan before slicing. Store in an airtight bag for up to 3 days.

Olives, one of the oldest known foods, are believed to have originated in Crete as far back as perhaps 7,000 years ago. This Mediterranean staple is a good source of iron and copper, is high in antioxidants, and has anti-inflammatory properties that benefit heart health. Their high concentration of monounsaturated fats, especially when combined with their vitamin E content, are thought to exert a protective effect on the body's cells, lowering inflammation in the body's tissues. These anti-inflammatory properties may help lessen the severity of asthma, osteoarthritis, and rheumatoid arthritis.

DESSERTS

Where would celebrations be without sweets? We are used to colossal cakes for birthdays, pies and cookies for holidays, and plenty of ice cream for summer fun. Unfortunately, this bonanza of refined sugar is doing no favors for your health or longevity. While I am against excessive sugar and food with no nutrition, I heartily believe there is room for dessert at the table. Personally, I eat a bowl of mouthwatering mixed berries with soy yogurt drizzled on top almost every night.

Here you will find a small selection of yummy deserts that are a sweet ending to any meal and also a boon for longevity. When studying centenarians, I noticed that they did indeed eat sweets after dinner, usually fruit, but they waited about a half an hour after dinner to indulge. I recommend you do the same, to give your digestion time to process your last meal before laying on the sweets. *Bon appétit!*

BERRYLICIOUS AND DELICIOUS!

BENEFITS: HEART + IMMUNITY + BRAIN & VISION

This is a dessert I could eat every night! I don't eat dairy and I try to avoid sugar, so when I am out with friends, I leave the chocolate cake to them and order a bowl of berries. Just about every restaurant has berries to offer, which they usually use for garnish, but they always bring it for me without a problem. Chock-full of vitamin C, fiber, antioxidants, and natural sweetness, these free-radical fighters make the perfect dessert.

SERVES 4

½ cup strawberries, hulled and halved

½ cup blueberries

½ cup blackberries

½ cup raspberries

1 tablespoon finely grated orange zest

A small bunch of fresh mint, chopped

Lowfat, unsweetened yogurt, for serving

1. Mix the strawberries, blueberries, blackberries, raspberries, orange zest, and mint gently in a serving bowl until combined.

2. Serve the fruit in bowls with a few dollops of yogurt for a refreshing summertime treat!

In Chinese medicine, red foods like **strawberries** are thought to be supportive of the heart-small intestine network. Indeed, the strawberry's content of folate, fiber, high antioxidants and phytochemicals are an ideal combination for heart health. Like blueberries, antioxidant-filled strawberries are supportive of neurological function. And just one serving, about eight strawberries, provides more vitamin C than an orange. Choose organic whenever possible to protect yourself from the high pesticide levels in conventionally grown berries.

PECAN PUDDING

BENEFITS: BRAIN & VISION

I fell in love with this pecan recipe when I was having dinner at the home of a friend. I begged for the recipe, and she eventually shared it with me. We can all benefit from her generosity in sharing, because this is one delectable dessert that is as healthy as it is mouthwatering! Pecans and walnuts have a similar highly nutritious profile; they are both brain foods, filled with beneficial fatty acids and also boasting a high protein content.

SERVES 4

2 cups soy milk
½ cup pecans or walnuts
¼ to ⅓ cup maple or brown rice syrup, or to taste
3 tablespoons arrowroot powder, kudzu powder, or sweet rice flour
2 tablespoons carob powder

1. Put the soy milk, pecans, ¼ cup maple syrup, arrowroot powder, and carob powder into a blender and blend until smooth. Pour the mixture into a small saucepan. Taste the mixture and add a little more syrup if you want it sweeter.

2. Heat the mixture over low heat, stirring constantly, until the pudding thickens and just begins to simmer. Immediately remove from the heat and serve warm.

A nutritionally very balanced food, **pecans** have a high content of iron, making them helpful for women. Pecans are full of phytosterols, plant compounds that decrease bad cholesterol in the body, and they provide 10 percent of the recommended daily amount of fiber, which also benefits cholesterol levels and aids in digestion. Additionally, pecans may help control high blood pressure, reduce risk of cancer, and defend against neurological disease. They can be a part of a weight management program, but don't eat more than a handful a day, as they are high in calories.

APPLE QUINOA CAKE

BENEFITS: HEART + ANTI-INFLAMMATION + DIGESTION

A patient of Mexican descent served this dish, her grandmother's recipe, at her home, and I enjoyed it so much that I asked for the recipe. The original used sugar and cream, so I adapted it to be gluten- and dairy-free. Quinoa, considered a sacred grain by the Incas, appears here in flour form, offering its high protein and excellent cardiovascular benefits. The apples are fiber-rich and full of vitamin C. A slice a day keeps the doctor away!

MAKES 1 CAKE

1¾ cups quinoa flour
1   cup dried cranberries
½   cup chopped walnuts
½   teaspoon baking soda
½   teaspoon baking powder
½   teaspoon sea salt
½   teaspoon ground cloves
1   egg, beaten
½   cup virgin coconut oil, plus more
     for greasing pan
2   large apples, peeled, cored
     and diced

1. Preheat oven to 350°F. Grease a 9-inch round cake pan.

2. Mix ¼ cup of the flour with the cranberries and walnuts in a small bowl and set aside. Put the remaining flour into a large mixing bowl and add the baking soda, baking powder, salt, and cloves; whisk to combine. In another bowl, whisk the egg and oil together until combined, and pour it into the flour bowl. Mix until just combined, and then fold the apples, cranberries and walnuts into the dough. Pour the batter into the prepared pan and bake for 45 minutes, or until a cake tester inserted in the center comes out clean.

3. Cool the cake for 10 minutes in the pan on a rack before inverting and cooling completely. Slice and serve.

Apples contribute to a healthy heart with their rich pectin content, which decreases cholesterol levels. Pectin also helps prevent colon cancer, one of the top causes of death in adults over age sixty. Additionally, apples reduce the risk of breast and lung cancer. A great source of vitamin C and peptides, apples support skin health. The apple peel is filled with antioxidant polyphenols, which protect you from free radical damage and unwanted inflammation in the body.

STEAMED HONEY-GLAZED ASIAN PEAR WITH LILY BULBS

BENEFITS: CLEANSING + ANTI-AGING BEAUTY

This recipe from China was created for the empress to preserve her beauty and her youthful complexion. Asian pears have a high content of copper, and lily bulbs contain a good amount of vitamin C and biotin, both antioxidants that are very supportive to the skin. All told, this dessert will help you put your best face forward for years to come!

SERVES 4

4   Asian pears
1   lemon, halved
½   cup local wildflower honey
½   ounce (15 grams) lily bulb powder
½   ounce (15 grams) dried lily
     bulb pieces
4   cinnamon sticks
     Seeds of ½ pomegranate,
     for garnish

1. Preheat the oven to 375°F.

2. Wash, peel and core the pears. Squeeze lemon juice all over them to prevent oxidation and put them in a shallow baking dish.

3. Using a pastry brush, coat the outside of each pear with honey, followed by sprinkling of lily bulb powder. Bake the pears uncovered until slightly browned on the outside, 10 to 15 minutes.

4. Meanwhile, set up a bamboo steamer basket over a wok or large skillet of gently simmering water. Transfer the pears to small serving bowls. Insert a cinnamon stick into the center of each cored pear and sprinkle some lily bulb pieces over each. Put the bowls in the steamer, cover, and steam until tender, about 10 minutes.

5. Carefully remove the pears from the steamer, garnish with lily bulb pieces and a sprinkling of pomegranate seeds, and serve warm.

Lily bulbs have been used medicinally for centuries. Even children in China know to use lily bulbs to relieve cough and mucus. They are used to help strengthen the respiratory tract, prevent coughs and colds, and induce peaceful sleep. You can easily find lily bulbs in Asian markets, herbal specialty shops, and online.

Asian pears, a cousin to the more traditional European pears, have brownish-yellow outsides and a juicy, crisp white center with a texture similar to an apple. Traditional Chinese medicine uses them to detoxify, quench thirst, relieve restlessness, promote urination, treat constipation, heal skin lesions, promote overall skin health, lubricate the throat, and relieve a cough. Asian pears are especially prized by Chinese herbalists as a way to eliminate dark circles under the eyes. With their content of copper, fiber, vitamin C, and other antioxidants, Asian pears are a nutritious snack.

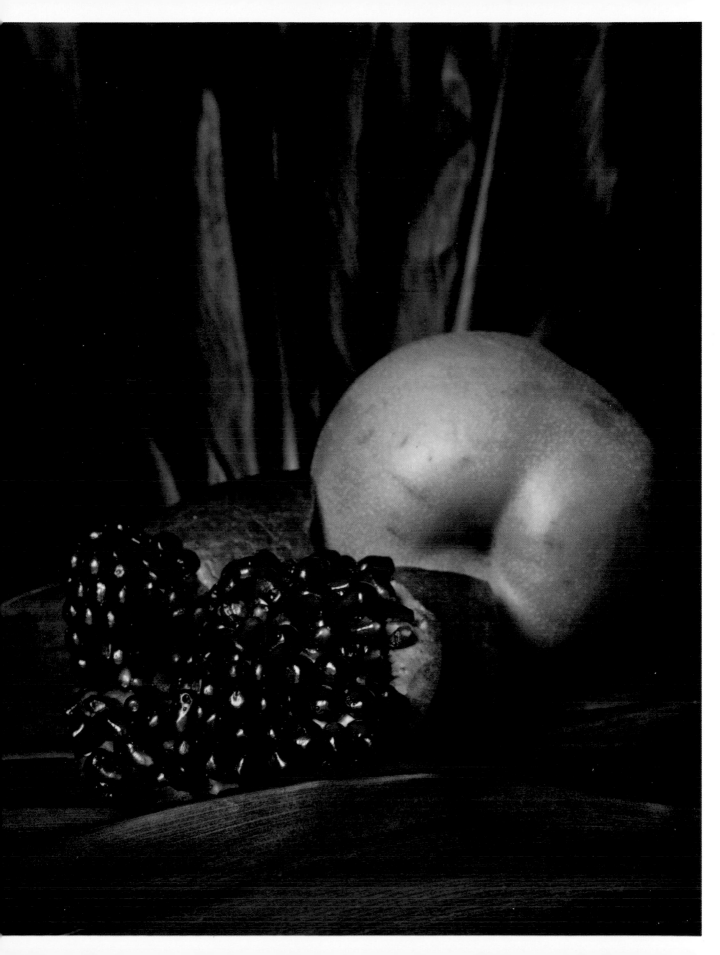

RESOURCES

Ask Dr. Mao

The official website for *Secrets of Longevity Cookbook* and Dr. Mao's other books. Ask Dr. Mao is a natural health search engine that contains thousands of searchable health questions and answers, as well as articles about health, wellness, and longevity. You may also look up and purchase Dr. Mao's health and herbal products. You can also sign up for his weekly e-newsletter.

www.askdrmao.com

Acupuncture.com

The oldest, most comprehensive, and most informative Web site on the Internet for acupuncture, Chinese herbal medicine, nutrition, tuina bodywork, tai chi, qigong, and related practices. This excellent resource for both consumers and practitioners offers access to hundreds of publications and herbal products.

www.acupuncture.com
info@acupuncture.com

American Academy of Anti-Aging Medicine

An organization with a membership of 11,500 physicians and scientists from sixty-five countries, the American Academy of Anti-Aging Medicine (A4M) is a medical society dedicated to the advancement of therapeutics related to the science of longevity medicine. Its Web site contains a wealth of research articles related to longevity and anti-aging therapeutics. It also conducts anti-aging conferences around the world.

www.worldhealth.net
info@worldhealth.net

Center for Food Safety

A nonprofit organization advocating for strong organic standards, promoting sustainable agriculture, and protecting consumers from the hazards of pesticides and genetically engineered food.

www.centerforfoodsafety.org
office@centerforfoodsafety.org

Gerontology Research Group

A group of professors, research scientists, and doctors sharing the latest findings as well as thought-provoking opinions on aging and life-extension techniques. Founded by Dr. L. Stephen Coles, MD, PhD, a professor and researcher in stem cell technology and longevity medicine at the University of California at Los Angeles School of Medicine, it also hosts monthly forums open to the public on the UCLA campus.

www.grg.org

The Grain and Salt Society

Offers unrefined sea salts, organic bulk whole foods, traditional cookware, hygiene products, and books.

www.celtic-seasalt.com
info@celtic-seasalt.com

Herb Research Foundation

Provides useful information on well-researched therapeutic herbs and publishes an herb magazine, *HerbalGram*.

www.herbs.org

Tao of Wellness

Health and wellness centers in Southern California that specialize providing quality service in acupuncture and Chinese medicine. Co-founded by Dr. Maoshing Ni.

1131 Wilshire Blvd., Suite 300
Santa Monica, CA 90401
www.taoofwellness.com
contact@taoofwellness.com

Whole Foods Market

Founded in 1980 as one small store in Austin, Texas, Whole Foods Market is now the world's leading retailer of natural and organic foods, with more than 170 stores in North America and the United Kingdom. These stores are a good place for healthy, mostly organic food, dietary supplements, and household cleaning supplies.

www.wholefoods.com

World Research Foundation

WRF established a unique, international, health information network to help people stay informed of all available treatments around the world. This nonprofit is one of the only groups that provides health information on both allopathic and alternative medicine techniques.

41 Bell Rock Plaza
Sedona, AZ 86351
www.wrf.org
info@wrf.org

Yo San University

An accredited graduate school of traditional Chinese medicine founded by Dr. Maoshing Ni and his family. Its rigorous academic, clinical, and spiritual development programs train students for the professional practice of acupuncture and Eastern medicine. Its ongoing community-based Healthy Aging Initiative is funded by a research grant from the Unihealth Foundation.

13315 W. Washington Blvd., Suite 200
Los Angeles, CA 90066
www.yosan.edu
admissions@yosan.edu

GENERAL RESOURCES

Anderson, James W. "Dietary Fiber and Diabetes." *Journal of the American Dietetic Association*, September 1987, 9:1189–1197.

Balch, James F., and Phyllis A. Balch. *Prescription for Nutritional Healing.* New York: Avery Publishing Group, 1990.

Barbul, Adrian, et al. "Arginine Stimulates Lymphocyte Immune Response in Healthy Human Beings." *Surgery*, 1981, 90:244–251.

"Be Your Best: Nutrition After Fifty." Washington, DC: American Institute for Cancer Research, 1988.

Borek, Carmia. *Maximize Your Health-Span with Antioxidants.* New Canaan, CT.: Keats Publishing, 1995.

Campbell, Ph.D., T. Colin and Thomas M. Campbell. *The China Study: The Most Comprehensive Study of Nutrition Ever Conducted and the Startling Implications for Diet, Weight Loss, and Long-term Health*. BenBella Books, 2006.

Caragay, Alegria B. "Cancer-Preventive Foods and Ingredients." *Food Technology*, April 1992, 46:65–68.

Cutler, Richard G. "Antioxidants and Aging." *American Journal of Clinical Nutrition*, 1991, 53:373S–379S.

"Diet and Cancer." American Institute for Cancer Research Information Series, 1992.

"Diet, Nutrition, and Prostate Cancer." American Institute for Cancer Research Information Series, 1991.

—. *The Green Pharmacy Anti-Aging Prescriptions: Herbs, Foods, and Natural Formulas to Keep You Young*. Emmaus, PA.: Rodale Books, 2001.

Evans, W. J. "Exercise, Nutrition and Aging." *Journal of Nutrition*, 1992, 122:796–801.

"Garlic, Tomatoes and Other Produce Fight Nitrosamine Formation." *Science News*, 1991, 145:190.

"Ginger and Atractylodes as an Anti-Inflammatory." *HerbalGram*, 1993, 29:19.

Gordon, James S. *Comprehensive Cancer Care: Integrating Alternative, Complementary and Conventional Therapy*. New York: Perseus Books Group, 2000.

Haas, Elson M. *Staying Healthy with Nutrition*. Berkeley, CA.: Celestial Arts, 1992.

"Herbs and Spices May Be Barrier Against Cancer, Heart Disease." *Environmental Nutrition*, June 1993.

Howell, A., et al. "Inhibition of the Adherence of P-fimbriated Escherichia Coli to Uroepithelial-cell Surfaces by Proanthocyanidin Extracts from Cranberries." *New England Journal of Medicine*. 1998: 339:1085–86.

Institute of Medicine. *Dietary Reference Intakes for Water, Potassium, Sodium Chloride, and Sulfate*. Washington, DC: National Academies Press; 2004.

Jenson, Bernard Anderson, and Mark Anderson. *Empty Harvest: Understanding the Link Between Our Food, Our Immunity, and Our Planet*. New York: Avery Publishing Group, 1990.

Johnston, Carol S., Claudia Meyer, and J. C. Srilakshmi. "Vitamin C Elevates Red Blood Cell Glutathione in Healthy Adults." *American Journal of Clinical Nutrition*, 1993, 58:103–105.

Keough, Carol. *The Complete Book of Cancer Prevention*. Emmaus, PA: Rodale Press, 1988.

Murata A., et al. "Prospective Cohort Study Evaluating the Relationship Between Salted Food Intake and Gastrointestinal Tract Cancer Mortality in Japan." *Asia Pacific Journal of Clinical Nutrition*. 2010: 19(4): 564–71.

Ni, Maoshing, and Cathy McNease. *The Tao of Nutrition*. Los Angeles: Seven Star Communications, 1993.

Pitchford, Paul. *Healing with Whole Foods*. Berkeley, CA: North Atlantic Books, 2002.

Sanchez, Albert, et al. "Role of Sugars in Human Neutrophilic Phagocytosis." *American Journal of Clinical Nutrition*. November 26, 1973: 1180–1184

Sun, Jian Ming, et al. *Secrets of Longevity throughout Chinese History*. Xian, China: Tienze Publisher, 1989.

Tucker, Don M., et al. "Nutrition Status and Brain Function in Aging." *American Journal of Clinical Nutrition*, 1990, 52:93–102.

U.S. Department of Agriculture, "Nutritive Value of American Foods in Common Units." *Agriculture Handbook No. 456*, 1975.

Walford, Roy L., and Lisa Walford. *The Anti-Aging Plan: The Nutrient-Rich, Low-Calorie Way of Eating for a Longer Life—The Only Diet Scientifically Proven to Extend Your Healthy Years*. New York: Marlowe & Company, 2005.

Weil, Andrew T. *Eating Well For Optimum Health: The Essential Guide to Bringing Health and Pleasure Back to Eating*. New York: Perennial Currents, 2001.

Werbach, M.R. *Nutritional Influences on Illness*. New Canaan, CT: Keats, 1987.

Yeager, Selene, et al. *New Foods for Healing*. Emmaus, PA: Rodale Press, 1998.

ACKNOWLEDGMENTS

My first thanks goes to my mother, who patiently and creatively fulfilled the picky palates of the three men in her life—my father, my brother, and me—while we were growing up. Watching and assisting her in the kitchen was a treat, as she worked with whatever ingredients were at hand and transformed them into delicious and healthy works of art.

Gratitude goes to the countless centenarians who allowed me into their homes and shared with me their favorite "longevity" dishes and also to the many patients who gave me their family recipes from long-living relatives.

I am lucky to have my wife Emm, whose culinary skills won me over and continue to wow those who get invited to dinner.

Special thanks to my dear friend and renowned photographer Phillip Dixon, whose masterful photographs brought the art out of food. I am also grateful to our masterful food stylist, Kate Martindale, who brought out the beauty in the recipes.

I could not have done this book without the patient and steadfast encouragement and support of my collaborator and designer-extraordinaire Laurie Dolphin, whose beautiful designs grace the pages of this book. I am equally grateful to Allison Meierding, whose ability to channel my thoughts into articulate language and visuals helped to make this material flow. There is no doubt that a book is a co-creation. I appreciate the expertise of Wesley Martin, our recipe editor, and the editing skills of Mary Grace Foxwell and Devorah Lev Tov. A notable thank you to Stuart Shapiro for his tireless support and vision in helping us grow *Secrets of Longevity*. Finally, my deep gratitude and appreciation goes to Chris Schillig of Andrews McMeel, who had the insight to take this project on and guide it to fruition and also to production editor Christi Clemons Hoffman, who pulled all the pieces together and kept everything flowing smoothly.

INDEX

A

alcohol, 9, 14–15, 26
almond milk, 13, 61, 62
almonds, 124
    Almond and Veggie Stir-Fry, 124
    Muesli Parfait, 73
    Vegetable Almond Pie, 126
aluminum cookware, 32
angelica root, 139
animal foods, 4, 38, 43, 44
    See also *specific types*
anti-aging foods, 8–9
    Anti-Aging Brain Mix, 159
anti-inflammation menus, 54–56
Anti-Inflammatory Spice Blend, 48
    Squash Peanut Soup, 88
antibiotics, 12, 15, 18
antioxidants, 14, 17, 34
apples, 17, 171
    Apple Quinoa Cake, 171
    Orange Fruit Salad with Maple-Glazed
        Ginger Pecans, 105
apricots, 64, 154
    Anti-Aging Brain Mix, 159
    Honey-Glazed Masala Chicken with
        Apricots, 154
    Hunza Brain Tonic, 64
    Muesli Parfait, 73
arthritis, 48
artichokes, 152
    Lemon Chicken with Artichoke Hearts,
        152
artificial sweeteners, 20
Asian herbs and spices, 28–29
    Eight Precious Herbs formula, 139
    spice blends, 47–49
Asian pears, 172
    Steamed Honey-Glazed Asian Pear with
        Lily Bulbs, 172
asparagus, 17, 85
    Asparagus-Zucchini Blossom Frittata,
        84–85
    Seaweed and Vegetable Medley, 121
avocado oil, 25
avocados, 17, 66, 161
    Avocado, Flax, and Coconut Smoothie,
        67
    Avocado-Goji Berry Smoothie, 66
    Avocado Hummus, 161
    Guacamole with Kale Chips, 164
    Mango-Avocado Salad, 111
    Quinoa Brown Rice Sushi, 134
    Savory Oatmeal with Pine Nuts,
        Avocado, and Egg, 74
    Warm Cod Salad, 113

B

baking, 45
baking soda, for cleaning, 36
bananas, 61, 106
    Banana Buckwheat Pancakes, 79
    Grapefruit Salad, 106

basil, 147
    Halibut Crudo, 147
    Stuffed Sardines with Pesto, 142
beans and legumes, 4, 8, 12, 23, 43
    Dr. Mao's Hot Herbal Cereal, 77
    Immunity Soup, 92
    Vegan Milk, 62–63
    See also black beans; green beans; *other*
        specific types
beef
    Spicy Tri-Color Pepper Beef with
        Himalayan Goji Berries, 157
beets, 91
    Immunity-Boosting Borscht with Porcini
        Mushrooms, 91
bell peppers, 144
    Asparagus-Zucchini Blossom Frittata,
        84–85
    Broccoli Stir-Fry with Yam Noodles, 123
    Seaweed and Vegetable Medley, 121
    Spicy Tri-Color Pepper Beef with
        Himalayan Goji Berries, 157
    Zesty Halibut in Soy-Ginger Dressing,
        144
berries, 29
    Berrylicious and Delicious!, 169
    See also *specific types*
beverages, 58–71
    alcohol and caffeine, 9, 14–15
    Dr. Mao's Honey Lemonade, 59
    Hunza Brain Tonic, 64
    Vegan Milk, 62–63
    White Grape Lemonade, 60
    See also smoothies; tea
BHA, 20
BHT, 20
bisphenol A, 23, 33
Black Bass with Coriander, 145
black beans, 9, 23, 63, 160
    Black Bean Hummus, 160
blueberries, 17, 61
    Anti-Aging Brain Mix, 159
    Banana Buckwheat Pancakes, 79
    Berrylicious and Delicious!, 169
    Energy Smoothie, 61
    Muesli Parfait, 73
borax, for cleaning, 36
Borscht, Immunity-Boosting, with Porcini
    Mushrooms, 91
BPA, 23, 33
brain health
    Anti-Aging Brain Mix, 159
    Brain and Vision Spice Blend, 49
bread
    Gluten-Free Olive Bread, 167
breakfasts, 72–85
    Banana Buckwheat Pancakes, 79
    Dr. Mao's Hot Herbal Cereal, 77
    Egg White Scramble with Chard and
        Porcini Mushrooms, 78
    Eggless Tofu Scramble, 80
    Muesli Parfait, 73

    Savory Oatmeal with Pine Nuts,
        Avocado, and Egg, 74
    Sweet Potato Crab Hash, 83
broccoli, 17, 123
    Broccoli Stir-Fry with Yam Noodles, 123
broth
    Cleansing Vegetable Broth, 87
brown rice. See rice
buckwheat, 79
    Banana Buckwheat Pancakes, 79
butternut squash, 101
    Chicken, Mango, and Butternut Squash
        Soup, 101

C

cabbage, 17, 137
    Cleansing Vegetable Broth, 137
    Creamy Cabbage, 136–37
    Vegetable Almond Pie, 126
caffeine, 9, 14
Cake, Apple Quinoa, 171
calcium, 11–12
calorie restriction, 38
cancers and cancer prevention, 11, 14, 23,
    38, 48
canned foods, 23, 25
cardamom, 153
carrots, 163
    Broccoli Stir-Fry with Yam Noodles, 123
    Curry Vegetables with Brown Rice, 133
    Quinoa Brown Rice Sushi, 134
    Soy Yogurt Dip with Carrots, Jicama, and
        Cucumber Sticks, 163
    Vegetable Almond Pie, 126
    Vegetarian Hot and Sour Soup, 89
cauliflower
    Almond and Veggie Stir-Fry, 124
    Creamy Sweet Potato Soup, 95
    Immunity-Boosting Cream of
        Mushroom and Cauliflower Soup, 94
celery, 17, 80, 128
celiac disease, 13
centenarian eating habits, 38–43
cereal
    Dr. Mao's Hot Herbal Cereal, 77
    Savory Oatmeal with Pine Nuts,
        Avocado, and Egg, 74
chamomile flower, 71
chard, 78, 148
    Cleansing Vegetable Broth, 87
    Egg White Scramble with Chard and
        Porcini Mushrooms, 78
    Miso-Glazed Sole with Swiss chard, 148
cherries, 43
chestnuts, 43, 129, 151
    Dr. Mao's Hot Herbal Cereal, 77
    Roasted Chestnuts and Wood Ear
        Mushrooms with Brown Rice, 129
    Sautéed King Prawns with Chestnuts
        and Figs, 151

chicken
   Chicken Leek Soup with Dried Plums
      and Quinoa, 99
   Chicken, Mango, and Butternut Squash
      Soup, 101
   Honey-Glazed Masala Chicken with
      Apricots, 154
   Imperial Chicken Infused with Eight
      Precious Herbs, 139
   Lemon Chicken with Artichoke Hearts,
      152
   Marmalade Chicken Brochettes, 153
   Spring Soup, 96
chickpeas, 161
   Avocado Hummus, 161
   Mint Pea Falafel, 138
chicory, 120
   Braised Chicory with Red Wine Vinegar,
      120
China Study, 4
Chinese wild yam, 100
   Chinese Wild Yam and Pumpkin Puree
      with Ginger, 100
chips
   Baked Sweet Potato Chips with Pumpkin
      Seeds, 166
   Guacamole with Kale Chips, 164
cholesterol, 6, 20, 24, 48
chrysanthemum flower, 70
cinnamon, 26, 145, 153, 154
citrus fruits, 6, 105, 153
   See also grapefruit; lemon; oranges
cleaning, 35–36
Cleansing Spice Blend, 48
   Summer Vegetable Soup, 97
Cleansing Vegetable Broth, 87
cloves, 145
coconut milk
   Avocado, Flax, and Coconut Smoothie,
      67
coconut yogurt, 13
   See also yogurt
cod, 113
   Warm Cod Salad, 113
coffee, 14
cold foods, 41–42, 104
cold types, foods for, 43–44
collard greens, 17
colorings, 20
condiments, 25–26
containers, 33, 34
convenience foods, 2, 3, 9
   packaged pantry items, 23, 25–26
cooking methods, 33–34, 44–46, 86
cookware and utensils, 30–35
Cool and Crunchy Salad, 108
Cool the Fire Tropical Smoothie, 69
cooling foods, 43
coriander, 145, 154
   Black Bass with Coriander, 145
   Coriander Spice Mix, 145
corn, 9, 17, 83

Summer Vegetable Soup, 97
Sweet Potato Crab Hash, 83
crab
   Sweet Potato Crab Hash, 83
cranberries, 8–9
   Apple Quinoa Cake, 171
   Grapefruit Salad, 106
crockpots, 34
cucumbers, 43, 108, 163
   Cool and Crunchy Salad, 108
   Soy Yogurt Dip with Carrots, Jicama, and
      Cucumber Sticks, 163
   Stuffed Cucumber Cups with Shiitake
      Mushrooms and Lotus Root, 118
   Warm Cod Salad, 113
Curry Vegetables with Brown Rice, 133
cutting boards, 35

D

dairy foods, 4, 9, 11–13, 43, 62, 117
   non-dairy alternatives, 24, 62–63, 94
dandelion, 87
   Cleansing Vegetable Broth, 87
   Immunity Soup, 92
dang gui, 139
deep-frying, 45
desserts, 168–73
   Apple Quinoa Cake, 171
   Berrylicious and Delicious!, 169
   Pecan or Walnut Pudding, 170
   Steamed Honey-Glazed Asian Pear with
      Lily Bulbs, 172
diabetes, 10, 14, 26, 48
digestion, 38, 39, 41–42, 104
Digestion Spice/Herb Blend, 49
dips
   Guacamole with Kale Chips, 164
   Soy Yogurt Dip with Carrots, Jicama, and
      Cucumber Sticks, 163
   See also hummus
dried fruits, 26–27
   See also specific types
dried mushrooms, 27
   See also specific types
drug interactions, 6, 47, 145

E

edamame, 112, 162
   Edamame Hummus, 162
   Edamame, Seaweed, and Tofu Salad, 112
Eggless Tofu Scramble, 80
eggplant, 17
eggs, 18, 43, 85
   Asparagus-Zucchini Blossom Frittata,
      84–85
   Egg White Scramble with Chard and
      Porcini Mushrooms, 78
   Savory Oatmeal with Pine Nuts,
      Avocado, and Egg, 74
Eight Precious Herbs, 139

   Imperial Chicken Infused with Eight
      Precious Herbs, 139
Emotional Tranquility Tea, 71
energy levels
   metabolism menus, 46–47
   Metabolism Spice Blend, 48
Energy Smoothie, 61
enjoying your food, 5–6, 10, 39–40
equipment, 5, 21, 30–35

F

Falafel, Mint Pea, 138
fats and fatty foods, 9, 15, 20, 24
   deep-frying, 45
   oils, 24–25, 45
fava beans
   Millet Pilaf, 131
fennel seeds, 145
fenugreek, 43
fermented foods, 12
figs, 151
   Muesli Parfait, 73
   Sautéed King Prawns with Chestnuts
      and Figs, 151
fish, 4, 18–19
   Baked Salmon with Lemon and Mango
      Salsa, 141
   Black Bass with Coriander, 145
   Halibut Crudo, 147
   Miso-Glazed Sole with Swiss chard, 148
   Saffron Ginger Fish Soup, 102
   Salmon Leek Salad with Ginger-Miso
      Dressing, 114
   Seared Salmon with Pickled Jicama, 140
   Stuffed Sardines with Pesto, 142
   Warm Cod Salad, 113
   Zesty Halibut in Soy-Ginger Dressing,
      144
fish oil, 25
Five Elements Powder, 61
flavorings, 25–26
flaxseed oil, 25, 50, 54
flaxseeds, 67, 162
   Avocado, Flax, and Coconut Smoothie,
      67
flours, gluten-free, 24
food colorings, 20
food preparation, 44–46
freezing foods, 29–30, 46
Frittata, Asparagus-Zucchini Blossom,
   84–85
fruits and vegetables, 4, 8–9, 16–17, 22, 43,
   44–45
   cleaning, 35–36
   eating organic, 17–18
   freezing, 29–30
   See also dried fruits; specific fruits and
     vegetables
frying, 44, 45

G

galangal, 102
garbanzo beans, 161
    Avocado Hummus, 161
    Mint Pea Falafel, 138
ginger, 43, 102, 153
    Chicken, Mango, and Butternut Squash
        Soup, 101
    Chinese Wild Yam and Pumpkin Puree
        with Ginger, 100
    Cleansing Vegetable Broth, 137
    Immunity Soup, 92
    Orange Fruit Salad with Maple-Glazed
        Ginger Pecans, 105
    Saffron Ginger Fish Soup, 102
    Salmon Leek Salad with Ginger-Miso
        Dressing, 114
    Spring Soup, 96
    Vegetable Almond Pie, 126
    Zesty Halibut in Soy-Ginger Dressing, 144
ginseng, 139
gluten, 4, 9, 13, 74
gluten-free grains and flours, 23–24
    See also *specific types*
Gluten-Free Olive Bread, 167
GMO foods, 13, 18, 148
goat cheese
    Grilled Portobello Mushrooms with Goat
        Feta, 117
    Mouthwatering Melon Delight, 107
goat's milk, 13, 117
goji berries, 66, 157
    Anti-Aging Brain Mix, 159
    Avocado-Goji Berry Smoothie, 66
    Dr. Mao's Hot Herbal Cereal, 77
    Spicy Tri-Color Pepper Beef with
        Himalayan Goji Berries, 157
Good Mood Spice Blend, 49
grains, 8, 23–24, 43
    See also *cereal; gluten; specific types*
grapefruit, 6
    Grapefruit Salad, 106
grapes
    Cool the Fire Tropical Smoothie, 69
    White Grape Lemonade, 60
grapeseed oil, 25
green beans
    Almond and Veggie Stir-Fry, 124
    Summer Vegetable Soup, 97
green tea, 9, 14
greens, 6, 12, 17, 36
    Cleansing Vegetable Broth, 87
    See also *specific types*
grilling, 44, 45, 117
    Grilled Portobello Mushrooms with Goat
        Feta, 117
Guacamole with Kale Chips, 164

H

Hainan Island, 69
halibut, 147
    Halibut Crudo, 147
Zesty Halibut in Soy-Ginger Dressing, 144
harmful foods, 9–15, 18–19, 20, 23, 24
Hash, Sweet Potato Crab, 83
heart disease, 11, 14, 38, 48
Heart Spice Blend, 48
    Asparagus-Zucchini Blossom Frittata,
        84–85
    Creamy Sweet Potato Soup, 95
    Stuffed Sardines with Pesto, 142
heart support menus, 50–52
hemp milk, 13, 62, 63
hemp oil, 25
hemp seeds, 62, 63
herbal teas
    Emotional Tranquility Tea, 71
    Internal Cleanse Tea, 70
herbs and spices, 27–29, 145, 154
    Dr. Mao's Hot Herbal Cereal, 77
    Eight Precious Herbs formula, 139
    spice blends, 47–49
    spice grinders, 35
high blood pressure, 11, 14, 20, 48
High Performance Powder, 61
honey, 26, 59
    Dr. Mao's Honey Lemonade, 59
    Honey-Glazed Masala Chicken with
        Apricots, 154
    Steamed Honey-Glazed Asian Pear with
        Lily Bulbs, 172
hormones, in animal foods, 12, 15, 18
Hot and Sour Soup, Vegetarian, 89
hot types, foods for, 43
hummus, 160
    Avocado Hummus, 161
    Black Bean Hummus, 160
    Edamame Hummus, 162
Hunza Brain Tonic, 64

I

immune function, 48
    immune support menus, 52–54
    sugar and, 10
Immunity-Boosting Borscht with Porcini
    Mushrooms, 91
Immunity-Boosting Cream of Mushroom
    and Cauliflower Soup, 94
Immunity Soup, 92
Immunity Spice Blend, 48
    Creamy Cabbage, 136–37
Imperial Chicken Infused with Eight
    Precious Herbs, 139
inflammation, 4, 10, 17, 24, 48
    anti-inflammation menus, 54–56
insulin resistance, 48
Internal Cleanse Tea, 70

J

jicama, 140
    Mango-Avocado Salad, 111
    Seared Salmon with Pickled Jicama, 140
    Soy Yogurt Dip with Carrots, Jicama, and
        Cucumber Sticks, 163

Vegetarian Hot and Sour Soup, 89
jujube dates, 92
    Immunity Soup, 92
    Imperial Chicken Infused with Eight
        Precious Herbs, 139

K

kale, 17, 164
    Cleansing Vegetable Broth, 137
    Guacamole with Kale Chips, 164
kefir, 12–13
kidney disease, 38
kitchen cleaning, 35–36
kitchen equipment, 5, 21, 30–35
kiwi fruit, 17
    Cool the Fire Tropical Smoothie, 69
kombu, 121

L

labels, reading, 19–20
lactose intolerance, 12
leeks, 114
    Broccoli Stir-Fry with Yam Noodles, 123
    Chicken Leek Soup with Dried Plums and
        Quinoa, 99
    Salmon Leek Salad with Ginger-Miso
        Dressing, 114
legumes. See *beans and legumes; specific
    types*
lemon, 59, 60
    Baked Salmon with Lemon and Mango
        Salsa, 141
    Lemon Chicken with Artichoke Hearts,
        152
    lemon peel, 153
    Marmalade Chicken Brochettes, 153
lemonade
    Dr. Mao's Honey Lemonade, 59
    White Grape Lemonade, 60
lettuce, 17
licorice, 139
lily blossoms
    Vegetarian Hot and Sour Soup, 89
lily bulbs, 172
    Steamed Honey-Glazed Asian Pear with
        Lily Bulbs, 172
liver function, 14
local foods, 16–17
lotus root, 118
    Stuffed Cucumber Cups with Shiitake
        Mushrooms and Lotus Root, 118

M

mango, 17, 101, 111
    Baked Salmon with Lemon and Mango
        Salsa, 141
    Chicken, Mango, and Butternut Squash
        Soup, 101
    Mango-Avocado Salad, 111
Maple-Glazed Ginger Pecans, Orange Fruit
    Salad with, 105
Marmalade Chicken Brochettes, 153

masala spice, 28, 154
    Honey-Glazed Masala Chicken with
        Apricots, 154
meal size and frequency, 3, 39, 50, 116
mealtimes, 39, 50
meat, 4, 15, 18, 20, 43
    Spicy Tri-Color Pepper Beef with
        Himalayan Goji Berries, 157
medication interactions, 6, 47, 145
Melon Delight, Mouthwatering, 107
menus, 50–57
    anti-inflammation, 54–56
    heart support, 50–52
    immune support, 52–54
    metabolism support, 56–57
mercury, 19, 87, 141, 142
metabolism menus, 46–47
Metabolism Spice Blend, 48
metal cookware, 31, 32
methylmercury, 19
microwaves, 33–34, 45
milk, 12, 117
    Vegan Milk, 62–63
millet, 131
    Dr. Mao's Hot Herbal Cereal, 77
    Millet Pilaf, 131
    Rosemary Millet with Yellow Split Peas
        and Zucchini Flowers, 132
mindful eating, 41
mineral supplements, 15
mint, 107
    Cool and Crunchy Salad, 108
    Mint Pea Falafel, 138
miso, 90, 148
    Miso-Glazed Sole with Swiss chard, 148
    Salmon Leek Salad with Ginger-Miso
        Dressing, 114
    Seaweed Miso Soup, 90
monosodium glutamate, 20
mood, 10, 13
    Good Mood Spice Blend, 49
Mouthwatering Melon Delight, 107
MSG, 20
Muesli Parfait, 73
multivitamins, 15–16
mushrooms, 78, 92
    Almond and Veggie Stir-Fry, 124
    Broccoli Stir-Fry with Yam Noodles, 123
    Curry Vegetables with Brown Rice, 133
    Egg White Scramble with Chard and
        Porcini Mushrooms, 78
    Eggless Tofu Scramble, 80
    Grilled Portobello Mushrooms with
        Goat Feta, 117
    Immunity-Boosting Borscht with Porcini
        Mushrooms, 91
    Immunity-Boosting Cream of
        Mushroom and Cauliflower Soup, 94
    Roasted Chestnuts and Wood Ear
        Mushrooms with Brown Rice, 129
    Seaweed and Vegetable Medley, 121
    Stuffed Cucumber Cups with Shiitake
        Mushrooms and Lotus Root, 118
    Vegetarian Hot and Sour Soup, 89

N

napa cabbage, 137
    Creamy Cabbage, 136–37
    See also cabbage
neutral foods, 43
nitrites, 20
nonstick pans, 32
nontoxic cleaning, 36
noodles
    Broccoli Stir-Fry with Yam Noodles, 123
nori, 90, 134
nutritional supplements, 15–16
nuts and seeds, 8, 22
    Anti-Aging Brain Mix, 159
    Muesli Parfait, 73
    Vegan Milk, 62–63
    See also *specific types*

O

oats, 23, 74
    Dr. Mao's Hot Herbal Cereal, 77
    Muesli Parfait, 73
    Savory Oatmeal with Pine Nuts,
        Avocado, and Egg, 74
    Sweet Potato Crab Hash, 83
obesity, 38
oils, 24–25, 45
Olestra, 20
olive oil, 24, 25
olives, 167
    Gluten-Free Olive Bread, 167
omega-3 fatty acids, 24, 67, 90, 113, 141,
    142
onions, 17, 128
    Almond and Veggie Stir-Fry, 124
oranges, 105
    Orange Fruit Salad with Maple-Glazed
        Ginger Pecans, 105
organic foods, 12, 17–18
osteoporosis, 11, 15

P

Pancakes, Banana Buckwheat, 79
pantry items, 5, 21–29
papaya, 17, 69
    Cool the Fire Tropical Smoothie, 69
Parfait, Muesli, 73
peaches, 17
peanuts, 9, 63, 88
    Squash Peanut Soup, 88
pears
    Creamy Sweet Potato Soup, 95
    See also Asian pears
peas, 17, 138
    Curry Vegetables with Brown Rice, 133
    Millet Pilaf, 131
    Mint Pea Falafel, 138
    Seaweed and Vegetable Medley, 121
    Seaweed Miso Soup, 90
    See also yellow split peas

pecans, 170
    Muesli Parfait, 73

    Orange Fruit Salad with Maple-Glazed
        Ginger Pecans, 105
    Pecan Pudding, 170
pesticides, 17–18
Pesto, Stuffed Sardines with, 142
phthalates, 33
Pickled Jicama, Seared Salmon with, 140
Pie, Vegetable Almond, 126
Pilaf, Millet, 131
pine nuts, 125
    Anti-Aging Brain Mix, 159
    Brown Rice with Pine Nuts, 125
    Savory Oatmeal with Pine Nuts,
        Avocado, and Egg, 74
    Stuffed Sardines with Pesto, 142
pineapple, 17, 69
    Cool the Fire Tropical Smoothie, 69
plant-based diets, 4, 5, 8
plant milk, 13
    Vegan Milk, 62–63
    See also *specific types*
plastic utensils and containers, 33
plums, dried, 99
    Chicken Leek Soup with Dried Plums
        and Quinoa, 99
porcini mushrooms, 78, 91
    Egg White Scramble with Chard and
        Porcini Mushrooms, 78
    Immunity-Boosting Borscht with Porcini
        Mushrooms, 91
pork, 43
portion sizes, 3, 38, 42, 43, 116
portobello mushrooms. See mushrooms
potassium bromate, 20
potatoes
    Curry Vegetables with Brown Rice, 133
pots and pans, 31–32, 34
prawns, 151
    Sautéed King Prawns with Chestnuts
        and Figs, 151
preservatives, 19, 20
processed foods, 4, 5, 9, 11
    canned foods, 23, 25
    reading labels, 19–20
    recommended pantry items, 23, 25–26
    See also *specific types*
prunes. See plums, dried
Pudding, Pecan or Walnut, 170
pumpkin, 9, 100, 128
    Chinese Wild Yam and Pumpkin Puree
        with Ginger, 100
    Stuffed Pumpkin, 128
    See also squash
pumpkin seeds, 166
    Anti-Aging Brain Mix, 159
    Baked Sweet Potato Chips with Pumpkin
        Seeds, 166
    Millet Pilaf, 131

Q

quinoa, 23, 99, 134, 171
    Apple Quinoa Cake, 171
    Chicken Leek Soup with Dried Plums
        and Quinoa, 99
    Quinoa Brown Rice Sushi, 134

R

radish, 108
    Cleansing Vegetable Broth, 137
    Cool and Crunchy Salad, 108
raspberries
    Berrylicious and Delicious!, 169
raw foods, 42, 43, 97, 104
restaurants, 42
rice, 133
    Brown Rice with Pine Nuts, 125
    Curry Vegetables with Brown Rice, 133
    Dr. Mao's Hot Herbal Cereal, 77
    Quinoa Brown Rice Sushi, 134
    Roasted Chestnuts and Wood Ear
        Mushrooms with Brown Rice, 129
    Stuffed Pumpkin, 128
rice bran oil, 25
rice yogurt, 13
roasting, 45
Rosemary Millet with Yellow Split Peas and
    Zucchini Flowers, 132

S

saffron, 102
    Saffron Ginger Fish Soup, 102
salads, 43, 104–15
    Cool and Crunchy Salad, 108
    Edamame, Seaweed, and Tofu Salad, 112
    Grapefruit Salad, 106
    Mango-Avocado Salad, 111
    Mouthwatering Melon Delight, 107
    Orange Fruit Salad with Maple-Glazed
        Ginger Pecans, 105
    Salmon Leek Salad with Ginger-Miso
        Dressing, 114
    Warm Cod Salad, 113
salmon, 141
    Baked Salmon with Lemon and Mango
        Salsa, 141
    Salmon Leek Salad with Ginger-Miso
        Dressing, 114
    Seared Salmon with Pickled Jicama, 140
salsa
    Baked Salmon with Lemon and Mango
        Salsa, 141
salt, 4, 9, 10, 11, 20
salt water, to wash produce, 36
sardines, 142
    Stuffed Sardines with Pesto, 142
Savory Oatmeal with Pine Nuts, Avocado,
    and Egg, 74
seaweed, 9, 27, 90, 112, 121
    Cleansing Vegetable Broth, 137
    Edamame, Seaweed, and Tofu Salad, 112
    Quinoa Brown Rice Sushi, 134

    Seaweed and Vegetable Medley, 121
    Seaweed Miso Soup, 90
    Vegetarian Hot and Sour Soup, 89
seeds. *See* nuts and seeds; *specific types*
sesame oil, 25
sesame seeds and tahini, 9, 126
    Anti-Aging Brain Mix, 159
    Avocado Hummus, 161
    Black Bean Hummus, 160
    Dr. Mao's Hot Herbal Cereal, 77
    Vegetable Almond Pie, 126
Sexual Health Spice Blend, 49
sheep's milk, 13, 117
shiitake mushrooms, 9, 27, 92, 118, 136
    Cleansing Vegetable Broth, 137
    Immunity-Boosting Cream of
        Mushroom and Cauliflower Soup, 94
    Stuffed Cucumber Cups with Shiitake
        Mushrooms and Lotus Root, 118
    Vegetarian Hot and Sour Soup, 89
shopping tips, 16–17, 30
Skin Beauty Spice/Herb Blend, 49
slow cookers, 34
small dishes, 116–57
    Almond and Veggie Stir-Fry, 124
    Baked Salmon with Lemon and Mango
        Salsa, 141
    Black Bass with Coriander, 145
    Braised Chicory with Red Wine Vinegar,
        120
    Broccoli Stir-Fry with Yam Noodles, 123
    Brown Rice with Pine Nuts, 125
    Creamy Cabbage, 136–37
    Curry Vegetables with Brown Rice, 133
    Grilled Portobello Mushrooms with
        Goat Feta, 117
    Halibut Crudo, 147
    Honey-Glazed Masala Chicken with
        Apricots, 154
    Imperial Chicken Infused with Eight
        Precious Herbs, 139
    Lemon Chicken with Artichoke Hearts,
        152
    Marmalade Chicken Brochettes, 153
    Millet Pilaf, 131
    Mint Pea Falafel, 138
    Miso-Glazed Sole with Swiss chard, 148
    Quinoa Brown Rice Sushi, 134
    Roasted Chestnuts and Wood Ear
        Mushrooms with Brown Rice, 129
    Rosemary Millet with Yellow Split Peas
        and Zucchini Flowers, 132
    Sautéed King Prawns with Chestnuts
        and Figs, 151
    Seared Salmon with Pickled Jicama, 140
    Seaweed and Vegetable Medley, 121
    Spicy Tri-Color Pepper Beef with
        Himalayan Goji Berries, 157
    Stuffed Cucumber Cups with Shiitake
        Mushrooms and Lotus Root, 118
    Stuffed Sardines with Pesto, 142
    Vegetable Almond Pie, 126
    Zesty Halibut in Soy-Ginger Dressing,
        144

smoke point of oils, 25, 45
smoothies
    Avocado, Flax, and Coconut Smoothie,
        67
    Avocado-Goji Berry Smoothie, 66
    Cool the Fire Tropical Smoothie, 69
    Energy Smoothie, 61
snacks, 41, 158–67
    Anti-Aging Brain Mix, 159
    Avocado Hummus, 161
    Baked Sweet Potato Chips with Pumpkin
        Seeds, 166
    Black Bean Hummus, 160
    Edamame Hummus, 162
    Gluten-Free Olive Bread, 167
    Guacamole with Kale Chips, 164
    Soy Yogurt Dip with Carrots, Jicama, and
        Cucumber Sticks, 163
sodium, 4, 9, 10, 11, 20
Sole, Miso-Glazed, with Swiss chard, 148
soups, 43, 86–103
    Chicken Leek Soup with Dried Plums
        and Quinoa, 99
    Chicken, Mango, and Butternut Squash
        Soup, 101
    Chinese Wild Yam and Pumpkin Puree
        with Ginger, 100
    Cleansing Vegetable Broth, 87
    Creamy Sweet Potato Soup, 95
    Immunity-Boosting Borscht with Porcini
        Mushrooms, 91
    Immunity-Boosting Cream of
        Mushroom and Cauliflower Soup, 94
    Immunity Soup, 92
    Imperial Chicken Infused with Eight
        Precious Herbs, 139
    Saffron Ginger Fish Soup, 102
    Seaweed Miso Soup, 90
    Spring Soup, 96
    Squash Peanut Soup, 88
    Summer Vegetable Soup, 97
    Vegetarian Hot and Sour Soup, 89
soy and soybeans, 80, 148
    Edamame Hummus, 162
    Edamame, Seaweed, and Tofu Salad, 112
    Zesty Halibut in Soy-Ginger Dressing,
        144
    See also miso; tofu
soy milk, 13
soy yogurt, 13, 163
    See also yogurt
spice blends, 47–49
spice grinders, 35
spices. *See* herbs and spices; *specific types*
spinach
    Avocado, Flax, and Coconut Smoothie,
        67
split peas. *See* yellow split peas
Spring Soup, 96
squash, 88
    Chicken, Mango, and Butternut Squash
        Soup, 101
    Chinese Wild Yam and Pumpkin Puree
        with Ginger, 100

Squash Peanut Soup, 88
Stuffed Pumpkin, 128
squash, summer
Almond and Veggie Stir-Fry, 124
See also zucchini
star anise, 145
steaming, 44
stevia, 26
stir-frying, 44, 45
Almond and Veggie Stir-Fry, 124
Broccoli Stir-Fry with Yam Noodles, 123, 124
Sautéed King Prawns with Chestnuts and Figs, 151
Spicy Tri-Color Pepper Beef with Himalayan Goji Berries, 157
strawberries, 17, 169
Berrylicious and Delicious!, 169
Muesli Parfait, 73
Stuffed Pumpkin, 128
sugar, 4, 9, 10–11, 20
Summer Vegetable Soup, 97
sunflower seeds
Cool and Crunchy Salad, 108
Muesli Parfait, 73
supplements, 15–16
Sushi, Quinoa Brown Rice, 134
sweet potatoes, 9, 17, 95
Almond and Veggie Stir-Fry, 124
Baked Sweet Potato Chips with Pumpkin Seeds, 166
Creamy Sweet Potato Soup, 95
Sweet Potato Crab Hash, 83
sweeteners, 11, 20, 26
See also honey; sugar
sweets, 41
See also desserts
Swiss chard. *See* chard

T

tea, 9, 14, 43
Emotional Tranquility Tea, 71
Internal Cleanse Tea, 70
time-saving tips, 34, 45, 46
tofu, 80
Creamy Cabbage, 136–37
Curry Vegetables with Brown Rice, 133
Edamame, Seaweed, and Tofu Salad, 112
Eggless Tofu Scramble, 80
Quinoa Brown Rice Sushi, 134
Seaweed Miso Soup, 90
Spring Soup, 96
Vegetarian Hot and Sour Soup, 89
tomatoes, 17, 80, 137
Eggless Tofu Scramble, 80
Summer Vegetable Soup, 97
Warm Cod Salad, 113
traditional Chinese medicine
eating for your type, 43–44
resources, 174, 175, 176
trans fats, 20
turmeric, 145
turnips
Vegetable Almond Pie, 126

U

unhealthy foods, 9–15, 18–19, 20, 23, 24
utensils and cookware, 30–35

V

Vegan Milk, 62–63
vegetables
Broccoli Stir-Fry with Yam Noodles, 123
Cleansing Vegetable Broth, 87
Curry Vegetables with Brown Rice, 133
Seaweed and Vegetable Medley, 121
Summer Vegetable Soup, 97
Vegetable Almond Pie, 126
See also fruits and vegetables; stir-frying; *specific vegetables*
Vegetarian Hot and Sour Soup, 89
vinegar, 25–26
cleaning with, 36
vision health
Brain and Vision Spice Blend, 49
vitamin supplements, 15–16
vitamins, in dried or frozen foods, 27, 29

W

wakame, 112
walnut oil, 25
walnuts, 9, 159, 170
Anti-Aging Brain Mix, 159
Apple Quinoa Cake, 171
Muesli Parfait, 73
Walnut Pudding, 170
warming foods, 43–44
watercress, 96
Cleansing Vegetable Broth, 137
Spring Soup, 96
watermelon, 17, 43
Mouthwatering Melon Delight, 107
weekly menus, 50–57
wheat, 13
White Grape Lemonade, 60
wild yam. *See* Chinese wild yam
wine, 14–15, 26
winter squash. *See* squash
wood ear mushrooms, 89, 129
Roasted Chestnuts and Wood Ear Mushrooms with Brown Rice, 129
Vegetarian Hot and Sour Soup, 89

Y

yams and yam noodles, 123
Broccoli Stir-Fry with Yam Noodles, 123
yellow split peas, 132
Rosemary Millet with Yellow Split Peas and Zucchini Flowers, 132
yogurt, 12–13, 73
Cool and Crunchy Salad, 108
Energy Smoothie, 61
Muesli Parfait, 73
Orange Fruit Salad with Maple-Glazed Ginger Pecans, 105
Soy Yogurt Dip with Carrots, Jicama, and Cucumber Sticks, 163

Z

zucchini
Almond and Veggie Stir-Fry, 124
Broccoli Stir-Fry with Yam Noodles, 123
Summer Vegetable Soup, 97
zucchini flowers
Asparagus-Zucchini Blossom Frittata, 84–85
Rosemary Millet with Yellow Split Peas and Zucchini Flowers, 132

*May you live long,
live strong, and live happy!*